# FIX IT
## WITH
# FOOD

*Praise for the book*

A wonderful, well-researched compilation of health foods that can help save your body and soul. Must read.

–Kunal Kapur, Celebrity chef

Written in Kavita's typical refreshing, non-preachy style, the book is easy to read, filled with simple and practical tips, and can persuade anyone and everyone to begin eating more of these everyday superfoods. Read it!

–Navni Parihar, Actor

From bottle gourd to bananas, Kavita Devgan teases out the secrets of superfoods in simple, easy-to-digest prose. Read, eat and be happy.

–Shoba Narayan, Author

Whether for disease management, weight loss or longevity, we are continuously bombarded with expensive, fancy dietary advice. Kavita Devgan has drawn on our traditional wisdom and embellished it with modern scientific knowledge to tell us the truth about healthy foods, in her usual lucid style. Her suggestions are simple, accessible and inexpensive. Recommended reading!

–Dr Ambrish Mithal,
Chairman and Head of Endocrinology and
Diabetes at Max Healthcare

This book is truly a unique treasure trove of well-researched, intelligently expressed and balanced information about 'eating healthy' to 'stay healthy'. A must-read for all for your own well-being.

–Prof. (Dr) Ashok Seth,
Chairman, Fortis Escorts Heart Institute,
Padma Bhushan and Padma Shri Awardee

# FIX IT WITH FOOD

**SUPERFOODS TO BECOME SUPER HEALTHY**

# KAVITA DEVGAN

RUPA

Published by
Rupa Publications India Pvt. Ltd 2020
7/16, Ansari Road, Daryaganj
New Delhi 110002

*Sales centres:*
Allahabad Bengaluru Chennai
Hyderabad Jaipur Kathmandu
Kolkata Mumbai

Copyright © Kavita Devgan 2020

The views and opinions expressed in this book
are the author's own and the facts are as reported by her
which have been verified to the extent possible,
and the publishers are not in any way liable for the same.

All rights reserved.

No part of this publication may be reproduced, transmitted,
or stored in a retrieval system, in any form or by any means,
electronic, mechanical, photocopying, recording or otherwise,
without the prior permission of the publisher.

ISBN: 978-93-89967-07-4

First impression 2020

10 9 8 7 6 5 4 3 2 1

The moral right of the author has been asserted.

Printed at HT Media Ltd, Gr. Noida

This book is sold subject to the condition that it shall not,
by way of trade or otherwise, be lent, resold, hired out, or otherwise
circulated, without the publisher's prior consent, in any form of binding
or cover other than that in which it is published.

*To Dadu Papa and Beeji*
*And all our elders*

# CONTENTS

Foreword — xi
Introduction — xiii
How This Book Works — xvii

## PART 1
## THE SUPERFOODS

1. Apple — 3
2. Banana — 8
3. Beetroot — 13
4. Bell Pepper — 17
   Mini Chapter I: Easy-breezy Fixes — 20
5. Black-eyed Pea — 23
6. Bottle Gourd — 27
7. Carrot — 31
8. Cashew — 35
   Mini Chapter II: Beat the Bloat — 38
9. Cauliflower — 39
10. Chickpea — 43
11. Corn — 46
12. Custard Apple — 50
    Mini Chapter III: Disease Busters — 54
13. Date — 58
14. Eggplant — 63
15. Poha — 66
16. Fox Nut — 70
    Mini Chapter IV: Easy Hacks — 74
17. Ghee — 79

| | | |
|---|---|---|
| 18. | Green Gram | 83 |
| 19. | Guava | 88 |
| 20. | Indian Gooseberry | 91 |
| | *Mini Chapter V: Fix Estrogen Imbalance* | 95 |
| 21. | Jackfruit | 96 |
| 22. | Mango | 100 |
| 23. | Moringa | 104 |
| 24. | Mushroom | 108 |
| | *Mini Chapter VI: Sleep Better* | 112 |
| 25. | Orange | 113 |
| 26. | Papaya | 116 |
| 27. | Peanut | 121 |
| 28. | Pear | 124 |
| | *Mini Chapter VII: Hangover Cures* | 127 |
| 29. | Pineapple | 128 |
| 30. | Potato | 132 |
| 31. | Pumpkin | 136 |
| 32. | Radish | 141 |
| | *Mini Chapter VIII: Pollution Antidotes* | 146 |
| 33. | Sattu | 147 |
| 34. | Spinach | 150 |
| 35. | Sweet Lime | 155 |
| 36. | Sweet Potato | 159 |
| | *Mini Chapter IX: Lose It* | 163 |
| 37. | Walnut | 165 |
| 38. | Water Chestnut | 169 |
| 39. | Watermelon | 172 |
| 40. | Yoghurt | 176 |
| | *Mini Chapter X: Stay Cool* | 182 |

## PART 2
## 10 TOOLS:
## FOODS TO HELP YOU BECOME HEALTHIER

| | | |
|---|---|---|
| I. | 10 Peels That You Must Eat | 185 |
| II. | 5 Ancient Grains to Get Back on Our Plate ASAP | 189 |
| III. | 5 Summer Coolers | 194 |
| IV. | 7 Stay-happy Foods | 196 |
| V. | 7 Foods That Help Correct Hormonal Imbalance | 200 |
| VI. | 8 Indian Berries We All Must Eat | 203 |
| VII. | 8 Healthy-hair Foods | 207 |
| VIII. | 8 Wow-skin Foods | 210 |
| IX. | 13 Easy Foods That Can Help Save You From Pollution | 213 |
| X. | 15 Super Condiments | 216 |

## PART 3
## 40 DELICIOUS RECIPES

| | | |
|---|---|---|
| I. | Magnificent Mains | 225 |
| II. | Breads and Grains | 227 |
| III. | Snack Attack | 231 |
| IV. | Healthy Desserts | 232 |
| V. | Spectacular Sides | 233 |

Acknowledgements     237

# FOREWORD

A balanced diet delivering the nutrition needed for nurturing sound physical and mental health is essential for one's well-being throughout their life. This is an axiomatic truth that most people recognize either through their scientific knowledge or sheer common sense. However, understanding nutrition science and applying it to our daily habits becomes a daunting task when contradictory claims and rebuttals, all emanating from published research, seem to shake our beliefs on a daily basis. Where then do we look to for help in guiding our choices?

Kavita Devgan's book makes the task simple for us through a listing of superfoods whose value is backed by sound science. It also aligns with traditional wisdom, which prefers the holistic approach of consuming whole and wholesome foods to a reductionist approach of pumping single nutrients separately packed in pills or pouches.

The pitfalls of a narrow tubular vision, which often restricted nutrition research, became abundantly clear when a number of antioxidant vitamins (such as vitamins C and E, and beta-carotene) were tried as solo supplements to prevent heart disease and cancer. This was based on the observation that people whose diets were rich in such antioxidants had a lower risk of these deadly diseases. It was naively assumed that supplementing these protective nutrients as single supplements would provide the same protective effect. However, the supplementation trials failed ingloriously in demonstrating protection. That is, because single-nutrient supplements do not replicate the interactions of the many phytonutrients that are power-packed together in natural plant foods. Also, a pill taken at breakfast may not provide protection against unhealthy foods consumed at dinner. Ideally every meal should be balanced in composition. The fact that these trials failed does not mean that antioxidants are not protective—merely that they are best consumed directly from plant sources where they occur in the natural form and keep company with other nutrients in the right balance. This is increasingly being proven by scientific studies that evaluate the benefits of natural food items and composite diets. Score a big win for nature!

The report, Food in the Anthropocene: the EAT–*Lancet* Commission on healthy diets from sustainable food systems, released in 2019, strongly recommended predominantly plant-based diets as best-suited for human health as well as ecological sustainability. This is sound advice. Among plant foods, there are some that are especially beneficial, because they are power-packed with multiple protective nutrients. This book provides a list of those superfoods, with clear descriptions of their nutrient strengths and potential range of health benefits.

Kavita's talent lies in making the book an engaging read, with scientific facts conveyed in an easily comprehensible manner. Many persons who would have been deterred by the mention of diet (in their minds, DIET stands for 'Dare I Eat That') will shed their apprehensions and begin to believe that healthy eating can be pleasurable too. Such eating need not be complicated or faddist. All the benefits can be accrued through natural superfoods! Even for others who have a natural curiosity about healthy foods and frequently wonder about what to eat to protect their health, this book will give food for thought as they indulge in thought for food. Relish the book—it is a superfood for your brain.

–K. Srinath Reddy
President, Public Health Foundation of India

# INTRODUCTION

What are superfoods?

The whole idea of superfoods is a little vague. The word is thrown about a lot, and rather arbitrarily, and is today in almost every conversation that we have.

So I decided to google the word 'superfood', and surprisingly, the search threw up more results than even for the word 'dieting'. I find Google to be an apt and easy window to look into trends. It can tell you a lot about where the world is moving, what people are thinking and what trends they are leaving behind. So, this small exercise gave me hope that people are moving towards the right direction and thinking about the right things (I mean, superfoods instead of diets).

I have always believed that when you begin putting the right food on your plate—and by right food, I mean food that does something good for you—then calories take care of themselves and your weight issues get tackled on their own.

So, when you think about nutrition and not weight loss, you end up achieving both. Whereas when you focus on just weight loss, you lose some and then gain it all back and more! So, no good comes out of it.

This is where superfoods come in. The truth is that we are, in general, overfed, but our diet is unfortunately inadequate. Superfoods help fill that gap. Even though there is no one particular definition, and very often, the term is misused or simply used to market a product, it is still not very difficult to identify the actual superfoods.

For a food to be deemed as a superfood, it must meet

certain conditions: These foods deliver concentrated–extra large–doses of good-for-you nutrients like antioxidants, vitamins and minerals. Actually, almost every food is good for us in some way, but some foods deliver goodness in a huge quantity. They are so packed with nutrients that they work as potently as a medicine or a supplement, but of course, are far far better for us.

Here, it is important to understand that both nutrient density (lots of one nutrient) and diversity (many nutrients) are important markers for a food to be called 'super'. The diversity of nutrients as well as their richness in a food helps us determine its 'superness'.

The conditions to be a superfood don't stop here. Besides being rich in regular nutrients like B vitamins, calcium and protein, they pack a punch of antioxidants, phytonutrients and flavonoids as well. These healthy chemical compounds that exist in plants help build immunity, ensure longevity and prevent the onset of diseases. Some improve the regenerative capacity of our brain and others have the ability to reduce inflammation. For instance, oats contain beta-glucans, a component that helps lower cholesterol, while garlic (lahsun) contains allicin, which can strengthen our immunity. Pomegranate (anar), for example, contains ellagitannins (ellagic acid), with proven anti-cancer properties, while the Omega-3 in flaxseeds (alsi) is a great friend of our brain. Another such example can be the vitamin E in walnuts (akhrot), which are very heart-friendly. Do you get the drift now?

Once you have identified the superfoods, the next step is to draw the best out of them. There are rules for that too: You cannot compensate for a bad diet by eating one superfood a day. For instance, you eat an entire medium pizza one day and then immediately follow it up with a glass of wheatgrass juice. Sorry to break it to you, but that will not work in your favour. You need to fall in love with these superfoods and learn to pick them over other nutritionally empty foods, over and over again.

Also, you cannot focus on just one or two superfoods and forget about the others. No *one* food provides everything for everybody. A variety of nutrients help ensure that we are getting the nutrients we need for vital health and wellness. Variety is key here, as different foods deliver different benefits. Remember, the sum of what you eat is more important than any individual food.

We must also remember that expensive and exotic doesn't always mean that they are better. Quinoa is great for us and I write about its goodness often too, but if it is not available, then buckwheat and amaranth are equally good (and cheaper) options. Similarly, chia seeds are brilliant but then so are basil (sabja) seeds, and might even be more easily available. Kale is a beautiful addition to your diet nutritionally, but don't spend your entire life hunting for it when you can just incorporate more spinach in your diet.

When we are discussing superfoods, information is key. A 100 gm of sweet potato (shakarkandi) with the skin will give you 8.5 mg of beta-carotene, which is more than what kale provides (5.9 mg per 100 gm). It is agreed that blueberries are loaded with polyphenols (cancer-preventers), but you can get the same compounds from seasonal, indigenous berries, like jamun, phalsa, Indian gooseberry (amla), etc. and that too at a fraction of the cost of blueberries.

It helps to combine two to three superfoods together to multiply the benefits. For example, sattu (roasted gram floor) with coconut water makes the drink more potent, seeing as, along with protein from sattu, you get extra electrolytes and super-hydration through coconut water.

You must be aware of the form in which you are consuming the superfood. Often, they are so processed that they are of no use to the body. Many kinds of packaged super-juices—acai berry, noni fruit, pomegranate—can be high in added sugar. This beats the purpose.

## The Truth Is Simple!

What you eat greatly affects your health—both short- and long-term health. We live in an environment where we are bombarded with toxins, both tangible as well as those that are hidden and therefore, scarier. Pesticides and genetically modified organisms compromise our food, our air is polluted, and our water supply is a major source of concern. As a result, I feel, and rather strongly, that foods with the highest nutrient density are our best hope of enhancing our vitality in this rather toxic world we live in. My message in this book is nothing exotic or groundbreaking really—in fact, I am simply trying to reiterate the age-old, commonsensical eating habits that are steeped in ancient wisdom, and emphasize the one thing told to children by mothers since time immemorial: Eat your veggies.

And like them, I too would say that instead of looking for exotic, unparalleled sources of 'extraordinary nutrients', we should stick to the ordinary extraordinary foods that are easily available and accessible. This book, thus, is a compilation of foods that are a treasure trove of nutrients, and written with the hope that once you know how good they are for you, you would include them more in your diet, and gain from their goodness.

# HOW THIS BOOK WORKS

This book is a compilation of superfoods–the powerhouses filled with immense nutrients. There are three parts to this book.

Part I contains the major part of the book with 40 chapters in all. Each chapter will discuss the importance of one superfood, with emphasis on its benefits and why it should be included in your diet. It lays out in detail the importance of each food, the nutrients it provides and the multifarious ways it helps us. Most importantly, each chapter makes for an independent read and can be revisited as many times as you would like.

Besides, this part will also provide a total of 100 'Fixit' solutions to everyday problems in the form of mini chapters–from disease busters to pollution antidotes, foods that reduce your bloating, to foods that help you sleep.

Part II of this book includes certain tips and tricks for a healthy life. It contains the essential tools that can help you maintain a strong and healthy lifestyle in the toxic world we live in.

Finally, Part III of the book contains 40 recipes that are delicious and easy to make, and would help you on the path to a fitter you.

The idea of this book is to essentially reintroduce you to the foods that you are already familiar with, and also to introduce some new ones to you. It will remind you of their various benefits, helping you to incorporate them in your diet again. It will help you make a conscious effort towards a healthier body, a calmer mind and a satisfactory weight on the scale.

Note: All nutrition counts mentioned for the foods are approximate.

# PART 1

# THE SUPERFOODS

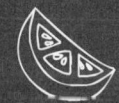

## Chapter 1

# APPLE

## An Apple a Day

The first thing I do when I sit for a food audit with my clients is to check how many fruits they are genuinely eating in a day. In most cases, they fall way too short of the advisable minimum of 2-3 servings a day. So, I try all tactics—persuading, cajoling, educating, often even frightening them to get them to eat more fruits. I am a firm believer in the important place that fruits have in our diet, especially when one is looking to gain health and lose pounds. And aren't we all! However, convincing my clients is anything but easy. People come up with excuses ranging from simple, honest ones like, 'I don't like their taste', to serious/complex ones like, 'My doctor has asked me to avoid raw foods', or 'I feel like a gas balloon after eating a fruit' (and not after eating that big juicy burger?). And my favourite to date—'My teeth are just not strong enough to chew fruits'!

I take the business of turning my clients and friends to fruit converts seriously, and have rarely failed to get them to make fruits a fairly important part of their diet. With fruits, variety is the trick—have them all by rotation to get the benefits of all. However, there are two fruits that I insist everyone must eat for sure and they are apples and bananas. Let me explain why I am so biased towards apples here.

Tell me what's not to love! They are crunchy (don't pick the overripe ones), sweet-tangy (a perfect mix, if you ask me), portable (I carry one in my bag every time I step out) and super-healthy too. We all have grown up listening to this oft-repeated saying: 'An apple a day keeps the doctor away.' Don't dismiss the saying because there is actually a lot of truth in it. We all know the basic qualities that make apples such an important fruit—they are high in fibre, low in calories, and flushed with vitamins and immunity-boosting antioxidants. Apples can also help ward off cancer, and prevent strokes and deadly heart attacks.

The nutritional stars in apples—fibre, flavonoids and fructose—work in tandem to keep us healthy. In fact, the fibre in apple packs a double punch and can help knock down cholesterol levels too, thus reducing the risk of the hardening of arteries, heart attack and stroke.

## More Good News

The happy news about apples does not end here. It has been found that ursolic acid present in an apple's peel can actually help you lose weight faster by increasing muscle mass and calorie burn. Now let us do the math: A small apple adds just 70 odd calories to your diet, so three of them will be close to 200 calories and will also provide 10 gm of fibre. Satiety plus weight loss—every weight watcher's best friend I would say! However, to get this benefit, you must have the apple with the peel (after washing it really well to get rid of the pesticides, of course) as ursolic acid is concentrated there. The vitamin C in apples is also present just below the peel.

## Your Pollution Antidote

If pollution is getting to you, then too apple will be a great helper for your lungs. Apples provide significant protection for the lungs because they contain high levels of antioxidant flavonoids called quercetin and khellin, which help open up the stuffed airways and protect the lungs from the harmful effects of atmospheric pollutants and cigarette smoke. What's more, eating quercetin-rich apples before you work out helps boost your exercise endurance by increasing the absorption of oxygen in the lungs. And this compound is known to cut the risk of stroke too.

### Beat Asthma

A high concentration of bioflavonoid (antioxidant) quercetin in apples has strong antihistamine, antioxidant and anti-inflammatory properties. Therefore, it is a known asthma-preventing food. Have the apple with the peel though, as most of the antioxidants are concentrated there.

> **Did You Know?**
> Malic acid in apples helps keep your skin firm, hydrated and pretty, and is a known fatigue buster too.

### That's Not All!

Apples contain a soluble fibre, pectin, which is truly the key to managing blood sugar and keeping insulin in check, therefore helping in keeping diabetes away. Also, apples derive almost all of their natural sweetness from fructose, a simple sugar, but one that is broken down slowly, especially when combined with the hefty dose of fibre provided by apples. Thus, this fruit actually helps to keep the blood sugar level stable.

Studies have shown that pectin helps lower bad cholesterol (low-density lipoprotein, or LDL) and increase the good cholesterol (high-density lipoprotein, or HDL). So basically, besides helping to keep you diabetes-free, apples take care of your heart's health too!

### Need More Reasons to Bite into an Apple?

They are great for your teeth; in fact, biting and chewing an apple stimulates the production of saliva in your mouth, reducing tooth decay. Also, they contain a high level of boron, which stimulates electrical activity in the brain and increases mental alertness. So, my simple advice is: Love them or hate—eat them!

### Easy Tips to Eat Apples

You can have apples in various ways—diced or thinly sliced in salads and cereals, as raw slices with an interesting dip, chopped in sandwiches, added to rice pilafs, or in stuffings and curries. Looking for an alternative to sweets? Try sliced apples and cheese, or with a nut (almond, peanut, walnut) butter.

### At a Glance

The benefits of eating apples include,

- Knocking down your cholesterol levels
- Saving your heart
- Protecting your lungs from pollution
- Losing weight faster
- Keeping blood sugar levels stable
- Reducing tooth decay

**Fun Fact**
Apples are mythology's favourite fruit. In the Bible, Adam and Eve, the first man and woman, ate this then-forbidden fruit in the Garden of Eden. In Greek mythology, goddess Eris uses a golden apple inscribed with the words 'To the Fairest One' to create tension among goddesses Hera, Athena and Aphrodite, which ultimately led to the Trojan War.

Chapter 2

# BANANA

### Go Bananas

Banana is considered an anomaly in fruits; apparently it is a fruit that leads to weight gain. The truth is far from it, actually. Bananas are, in fact, a slimming superfood. If you are looking for a proven way to satiate your hunger without gaining weight in the process, my advice is: Turn to the banana. First of all, it is a zero-fat food, and a medium-sized banana contains less than 100 calories. Secondly, it helps boost your metabolism and is loaded with resistant starch (RS), a kind of fibre that not just makes you full, but reduces those pesky cravings too. Not absolutely ripe but, firm, medium-sized bananas gives you 4.7 gm of RS, perfect to keep you full for long.

There are myriad benefits of bananas. Compared to an apple, a banana contains four times the protein, three times the potassium, and twice the carbohydrates, vitamin C, iron and phosphorous. What's more, a medium-sized banana contains less than 100 calories. Not bad at all!

It is important to note that RS consumption is also associated with lower cholesterol and triglyceride levels, and better calcium and magnesium absorption in the body. This translates to stronger bones and a heartier heart. It is small wonder then that the scientific term for banana is *Musa sapientum*, meaning 'fruit of the wise men'.

**Great Friend of the Gut**

The high fibre content of bananas facilitates digestion, thereby beating constipation effectively, without having to resort to laxatives. Bananas have a natural antacid effect in the body, so if you suffer from heartburn, try eating a banana for soothing relief. If had with a little salt, it effectively treats dysentery too. Plus, banana delivers the phytochemical fructooligosaccharide, which boosts the good bacteria in our colon and thus stops the bad bacteria from producing toxins that negatively affect our health. This compound also helps the body absorb important bone-strengthening nutrients like calcium and magnesium.

**Feel-good Fruit**

It's a happy fruit too. It's loaded with tryptophan, which gets converted into serotonin in the body, which boosts our mood, busts stress and makes us happier. In fact, a low level of serotonin is a known cause of mood disorders and depression. Bananas also rank as a feel-good food due to the high levels of tyrosine they contain, which is actually a precursor needed to produce the happiness-inducing neurotransmitters, serotonin and dopamine!

**Rock-a-bye Banana!**

Forget about the sleeping pill. If you are unable to sleep, just grab a banana. Its high magnesium, potassium and tryptophan content will lull you to sleep soon enough. Bananas also help the body naturally produce the sleep hormone, melatonin, due to its high vitamin B6 content.

## Hangover Cure

Bananas are a perfect fix for hangovers. It helps settle the stomach and ward off nausea because it functions as a natural antacid. The high dose of potassium in a banana also replaces lost potassium. For example, if you went to the loo way too many times last night, that not only dehydrated you, but also depleted the electrolytes in your blood: sodium, potassium, calcium and magnesium. The lost magnesium replaced by the banana will also help relax those pounding headaches by easing your distorted blood vessels.

## Get Going

Ever noticed that banana is a hot favourite with all athletes? That's because it delivers three natural sugars—sucrose, fructose and glucose—and an extra large amount of fibre. Therefore, it works on two fronts simultaneously—gives an instant energy boost as well as sustained and substantial energy (that's why you see so many top-level athletes munching on bananas during competitions). It also has a high iron content, so it has the ability to stimulate haemoglobin production in the bloodstream, and thus helps keep fatigue away.

### Did You Know?
Banana is a perfect 'rescue recipe' if you are trying to junk the cancer stick (cigarettes). The vitamins B6 and B12, and the high potassium and magnesium found in it help the body recover from the effects of nicotine withdrawal.

## Beat Asthma

Banana is one of the best sources of pyridoxine (vitamin B6), which helps beat asthma and also combats the physical effects of stress that the body goes through during an intense exercise session.

## Potassium Power

Banana is loaded with potassium—a mineral essential for keeping our blood pressure in check, for the nerves to function properly and also for promoting bone health. It also helps counter the high-salt diets (read: junk eating) that most of us indulge in, and saves us from the damage caused by them.

## Easy Tips to Eat Bananas

All said and done, if just biting into it is not really your idea of, let's say, a gastronomic delight (maybe you find them a bit bland), then just make the banana exciting. Banana for breakfast is a great idea. Take an oval dish and layer the bottom of it with a cup of cooked oats. Place one layer of horizontally sliced bananas over that. Now top this with another layer of oats, add a sauce of your choice and sprinkle some nuts. Or just make a banana smoothie with yoghurt or milk.

Reach for it in the late afternoon for a quick perk-me-up. Add it to a fruit salad, or have it spiced up. Peel a banana, lightly rub it with a mix of lime juice, honey and black salt. Let this rest for 5 minutes, and then enjoy your sweet-and-spicy banana.

Need a cooling snack? Try this: Peel a banana and dip it in yoghurt completely. Roll this in crushed cereal and freeze. Then bite in!

Move beyond the commonplace peanut-butter-and-banana sandwich drizzled with honey. Try instead a banana roti roll. Simply take a roti, smear it with peanut butter, place a banana on one side and roll it. Now, cut this into small discs and snack on it. Delicious!

### At a Glance

The benefits of eating bananas include,

- Keeping cravings away
- Taming blood pressure
- Cutting fatigue to size
- Stronger bones and a heartier heart
- Staying happy and depression-free
- Cleaning the gut

### Fun Fact
The first banana split was made in 1904, but bananas have been around much longer than that. Also interestingly, there is a red banana that tastes like raspberry, and another called the Blue Java banana, which tastes and feels like vanilla ice cream.

Chapter 3

# BEETROOT

### The Red-hot Solution for Everything

Have you ever tried beetroot buttermilk (chhaach)? It's super simple to make: Just puree 1 boiled beetroot in a mixer. Mix it with 1 cup yoghurt with 1 cup water and do a quick whisk. Next, heat ½ tsp oil, add ¼ tsp mustard seeds, 5–6 curry leaves, ½ tsp ginger (adrak) and 1 green chilly chopped finely. Add the tempering to the beetroot and yoghurt mix. Chill and drink.

But why am I promoting this delicious, if somewhat unusual, recipe?

That's because I am trying to entice everyone to incorporate more beetroot in their diet. I know the trouble with beetroot is that its unusual earthy taste takes some getting used to and therefore, it doesn't really find a place in our veggie shopping lists. But that needs to change. It is too good a food to not be eaten regularly.

### Your Heart's Friend

This red roughage is a good friend of our heart. Need convincing? Well, it has a very high nitrite content that gets converted to nitric oxide in the body. Nitric oxide helps dilate our blood vessels, leading to better blood flow. A glass of beetroot juice a day can actually help keep your blood pressure in check. Beetroot is also rich in anti-inflammatory antioxidant betaine, which helps keep our bad cholesterol levels down and also lowers homocysteine, a known risk factor for stroke and heart disease.

Yes, beets are that good, but we just don't eat them enough. Never have! 'Eat your greens', everyone never tires of saying. No one ever says, 'Eat your reds'. It's time to let the reds shine too.

### Beet That!

Beets are delicious, nutritious and low in calories (200 gm provides only 80 calories). Plus they are loaded with fibre—almost 6 gm of fibre per 200 gm of beet. They are a surprisingly good source of quality protein (200 gm of beet provides more than 3 gm of protein). It is also one of the richest sources of glutamine, an amino acid that is great for our intestinal health.

### Antioxidants Galore!

Beetroots have some vitamin C, a key antioxidant and immunity booster (and your answer to combat frequent cold and flu), as well as a mega dose of folate and potassium, both essential nutrients. Potassium also helps keep our blood pressure in check. Also, phytochemicals in beet assist in reducing the risk of breast cancer, besides helping prevent other cancers, such as of the lungs, stomach and colon. The flavonoids are one of the reasons for the deep red colour (which is why it is best to buy the deepest red ones you can) and help the body fight against free radicals, the harbingers of myriad lifestyle diseases and accelerated ageing.

### Detox, De-stress and Fight Dementia

Beets deliver betaine (also used in some depression medications), and tryptophan, both of which help us de-stress, feel happier and keep depression at bay. They actually work like chocolate, without delivering the fat. Betaine also helps trigger the detoxification and cleansing of our body and fight dementia by increasing blood flow to the brain.

### Did You Know?
Beetroot is great for beating a hangover. That's because betacyanin, another pigment that gives beetroot its colour, speeds up detoxification in the liver, which enables the body to turn the alcohol into a less harmful substance that can be excreted quicker than normal.

## Ancient Aphrodisiac

Beetroot was a popular aphrodisiac in ancient Rome. This is understandable as it contains high amounts of boron, a mineral that is essential for the production of sex hormones in humans.

## Easy Tips to Eat Beetroots

You can eat them raw, cooked or roasted. I usually simply grate them and add liberally to my salads and soups, or add chunks of them to a veggie stir-fry. Whatever you do, don't boil it and throw the water. If you do, you'll throw half the nutrients with that water. Instead, let the water cool, and then you can drink it.

Prefer the juice? If you find the beetroot's earthy flavour a problem, just squeeze some lemon into it. The sourness offsets the earthiness and adds a new dimension. You can also add some orange or lemon zest. Or add some apple juice if you prefer it sweeter. Like savoury? Spice up beet juice with fresh ginger or hot peppers.

You can even try this salad: Steam some beets, marinate them in lemon juice, olive oil and herbs of your choice, then roast them in the oven till they're done. Add some salad leaves of your choice, a few nuts (pine nuts [chilgoza] go well), and toss in a simple dressing of lemon, oil, black pepper and oregano. Chill and eat.

### At a Glance

The benefits of eating beetroot include,

- Saving your heart
- Detoxifying and purging toxins from the body
- Preventing lifestyle diseases and ageing
- Reducing the risk of cancers
- Busting your hangover

**Fun Fact**
Beetroots can be made into a wine that tastes similar to port.

Chapter 4

# BELL PEPPER

## Pep Up Your Health with Bell Peppers

A client of mine has been having a salad of bell peppers—all three: red, yellow and green—almost every second day before her lunch for the last few years. She loves their tangy taste. This way, inadvertently, she has been doing a lot of good to her body. Not many know that nutritionally loaded bell peppers are botanically a fruit with a taste that ranges from slightly sweet-tangy to hot. They are low in calories, and deliver vitamins A and C, potassium, folic acid, some protein and lots of fibre.

## The A to E Story

Bell peppers have a very high concentration of antioxidants. You need just one serving to cover your daily quota of vitamins A and C. The latter vitamin is great for our immune system, keeps your skin elastic and supple, and prevents arthritis. Vitamin A (beta-carotene) is anti-inflammatory and also good for our eyes. It also helps cut the risk of cancer by significantly reducing the free radical activity in the body.

Bell peppers also deliver vitamin E, which keeps our heart healthy, and vitamin B6, which keeps our nervous system ticking.

Significantly, red bell peppers deliver more nutrition (as they stay on the vine longer) compared to green bell peppers; they have almost 11 times more beta-carotene and 1.5 times more vitamin C.

## Weight Loss on Your Mind?

Sweet bell peppers have a compound called CH-19 Sweet. It resembles the capsaicin found in hot chillies and provides similar metabolism-boosting effects (and thus weight loss benefits). Plus, it doesn't burn the mouth and lips like capsaicin.

## There's More!

As mentioned before, bell peppers protect against cancer, thanks to their sulphur content. They also deliver lutein and zeaxanthin, which help protect the eyes from cataracts and macular degeneration. For this benefit, green bell peppers score better as they are one of the best natural sources of these antioxidants!

Finally, bell peppers are great for your brain's health too. They deliver vitamin B6, which increases the levels of serotonin and norepinephrine, leading to a better concentration level and a calmer mind. In fact, a low level of these chemicals has been linked to several mental health conditions like attention deficit hyperactivity disorder (ADHD).

### Did You Know?
Bell peppers contain traces of nicotine, which, in small amounts, is neuroprotective and helps lower the risk of Parkinson's disease.

## Easy Tips to Eat Bell Peppers

Now that's enough reasons—from preventing colds to cancer—to have more of these crunchy veggies, even if the taste takes a little getting used to. And if you don't like them raw, just steam them lightly as that actually boosts the efficacy of the antioxidants. However, as high heat may destroy some of the other nutrients found in bell peppers, best is to cook them lightly over slow heat and leave them crunchy.

I usually toss them into the pasta just before it is almost done. I love to eat them stuffed with myriad things like beans, rice, vegetables, cottage cheese, etc. Eat more of these; trust me you will love the crunch.

## At a Glance

The benefits of eating bell peppers include,

- Amassing lots of vitamins A, B-complex, E and C
- Gaining youthful skin and hair
- Boosting your brain's health
- Protecting your eyes from age-related degeneration
- Preventing Parkinson's disease

### Fun Fact
Besides the common green colour, bell peppers also come in red, orange, yellow, white and purple. There are black and brown bell peppers too, although these are difficult to find.

Mini Chapter I

## EASY-BREEZY FIXES

**Fixit Tip 1:** First step: Clean your house... and don't forget the fridge. When you have the 'wrong' food around, saying no is a difficult option. So, throw out the food that is not good for you.

Next step: Replace the junk with healthy, 'real' foods. Keep the good stuff around.

**Fixit Tip 2:** Make a list of the antioxidant-rich (vegetables and fruits), Omega-3-rich (flaxseed, walnut), high-fibre (whole grains), high-potassium (coconut water, sweet potato) foods... and go stock up today!

**Fixit Tip 3:** Clean eating does not mean giving up foods arbitrarily (dairy, wheat flour, carbs, fats). It just means eating a variety of food, with plenty of fruits and vegetables, and watching your overall calorie intake. No rocket science here. Just avoid falling for the fads.

**Fixit Tip 4:** If you don't want to worry about craving to go back for seconds, eat foods that are nourishing and packed with nutrients. Yes, I am talking about veggies and fruits.

**Fixit Tip 5:** Ever snacked on a plump piece of fresh coconut? Try it, it is supremely satisfying, super-delicious and every bite delivers health.

**Fixit Tip 6:** Don't skip lunch! Try this quick meal: Spinach and gram flour (besan) chilas with boiled potatoes, and sprouts chaat dressed with lemon juice. Eat with green chutney and flavoured yoghurt. It works because it is a perfect combination of carbohydrates and protein, with the goodness of veggies. Lemon juice has vitamin C, which helps absorb iron from spinach better. Yoghurt is a perfect add-on, as it is rich in probiotics and is low calorific compared to other dips.

**Fixit Tip 7:** Always shop for groceries alone and on a full stomach. With your mind free and stomach full, you'll make fewer impulsive (read: wrong) purchases.

### And Now for Some Easy-breezy Beauty Fixes:

**Fixit Tip 8:** To prevent sunburn damage, you need to score enough beta-carotene. It converts to vitamin A in the body, accumulates in the skin, and provides 24-hour protection against sun damage. Carrot (gaajar), pumpkin (kaddu) and sweet potato are great sources; in fact, 2 carrots a day can provide your daily requirement of beta-carotene.

**Fixit Tip 9:** Strawberries work at removing excess sebum (oily secretion) on your skin as well as nourish and revitalize it. They have strong anti-acne properties too.

**Fixit Tip 10:** Nectarines (shaftalu or aadu) have multiple bioflavonoids, which are great for our skin. The beta-carotene in them protect the skin from the harmful effects of UV radiations, and vitamin C contributes in collagen synthesis, keeping the skin youthful.

**Fixit Tip 11:** Chew on raisins (kishmish) to satisfy your sweet tooth and also score healthy and pretty-looking teeth and gums. Oleanolic acid, a phytochemical present in raisins, helps bust cavities and dental diseases. Also, the sugars it contains—fructose and glucose—are less likely to contribute to cavities than sucrose, the main culprit in oral disease.

**Fixit Tip 12:** Cherries deliver good skin by cleansing the blood, liver and kidney. They also detox by promoting regular bowel movements.

**Fixit Tip 13:** Figs (anjeer) are high in fibre and help to reduce constipation. They have vitamins B and C, phosphorus, potassium, and minerals like calcium and magnesium, which boost skin health. They contain some good fats too, which keep the skin well-moisturized and conditioned from within.

**Fixit Tip 14:** Litchi is loaded with antioxidant vitamin C, which helps slow down the ageing process and adds a glow to the skin.

Chapter 5

# BLACK-EYED PEA

### The Hidden Gem

Pulses (dal) are good for us and we all know that. Most South Asians have grown up eating dal in almost every meal, and now, even the United Nations (UN) has decided to highlight their benefits. In fact, the 68th UN General Assembly had declared 2016 as the International Year of Pulses. However, that said, the focus usually is always on a few kinds of dal—black gram (kali dal), red kidney beans (rajma), chickpeas (chhole) and sambar made with pigeon peas (toor dal)—and one unsung hero, black-eyed peas (lobia), always gets relegated to the background. In some countries, lobia are thought to bring good luck if eaten at the beginning of a new year, and so, are traditionally eaten on the first day of January. But I have friends who don't buy this anymore as part of their regular grocery shopping. It is extremely unfortunate I tell you, because the benefits they are missing out on are immense.

### Nutrients Galore

Not only are lobia low in calories (1 cup cooked lobia provides just 160 calories), they also deliver a high amount of fibre (8 gm) and are a fat-free food. They are also loaded with calcium, magnesium, iron (helps prevent anaemia), zinc and copper, besides being a powerhouse of protein (5 gm).

### The B Advantage

All pulses are a good source of folate, a B vitamin needed to form and maintain new cells—especially red blood cells—which are important to keep anaemia and fatigue away. This vitamin is absolutely essential for proper foetal growth, so pregnant women need loads of it. Lobia top the list amidst all pulses in the amount of folate they deliver. They also deliver a lot of another important B vitamin called thiamine, which helps maintain healthy nerves.

### Great-eye Peas!

Lobia deliver a lot of vitamin A, a vision-enhancing nutrient. This antioxidant is great for scoring healthy skin and boosting our immunity. It also helps protect our skin and mucous membranes.

> **Did You Know?**
> Lobia also delivers the hard-to-find trace mineral manganese, which protects the mitochondria, the structures inside cells that produce energy.

### Your Gut's Friend

Lobia are loaded with soluble fibre, which binds to cholesterol and helps throw it out of the body, besides protecting us from several intestinal disorders, and keeping constipation away. It helps keep your cholesterol levels healthy by preventing cholesterol from being absorbed into your bloodstream.

### A Weight Watcher's Friend

Fibre boosts satiety and that's why lobia are every weight watcher's friend. Their wonderful protein-and-fibre combination makes them a low glycemic index food (which means, they get used up slowly in the body, and don't lead to a surge in blood sugar), so they are good for losing weight and safe for diabetics too. Also, lobia contains a compound that acts as an amylase blocker; this delays the digestion of carbohydrates. So, basically, when you eat them with high-glycemic carbohydrates like bread, pasta and sugar, they help lower the glycemic index of the food and thus promote weight loss. That's why lobia-rice works so well.

### Your Heart's Friend

Getting cramps in your legs or feet? Foods rich in potassium (like lobia) are the first things to reach for. That's not all. The potassium in lobia is great to balance the excess sodium in our diets and keep our blood pressure sorted too, besides boosting our muscle strength and metabolism, and keeping the bones strong.

### Easy Tips to Eat Black-eyed Peas

There are more interesting ways to eat it besides just making a lobia curry. Think stews, soups, salads; in fact, lobia is very versatile and tastes well with almost all foods (potatoes and rice in particular) and that's why it is a delight to cook and eat.

Why not make a lobia salad by mixing them up with carrot, spinach, broccoli (other good vitamin A sources), and score a great dish for your eyes? Or a stew with some carrot, peppers and spinach?

## At a Glance

The benefits of eating black-eyed peas include,

- Improving your digestion
- Cutting down cholesterol
- Preventing anaemia
- Keeping your blood pressure down
- Boosting your eye health

### Fun Fact
Black-eyed peas get their name from their appearance; they are cream-coloured with a little black speck that resembles an eye!

Chapter 6

# BOTTLE GOURD

## Learn to Love the Bottle Gourd

I often go overboard with my love for the bottle gourd (also called lauki and ghiya) and on those days, the lunch menu often is channa dal with lauki, chilled lauki raita, and lauki peels and sprouts subzi to complete the lauki-special meal. Yes, this vegetable, so called as it looks like a bottle, is an absolute favourite. I love its sweet, mild taste and also the fact that it is so versatile.

## A Natural Coolant

Lauki is 96 per cent water and is inherently cooling; therefore, a boon during the summers. Also, it is loaded with potassium that keeps our blood pressure down and electrolyte balance sorted. It also prevents fatigue and is an effective detoxifying food that helps prevent nose bleeding during the summer months as well.

## Nutrition Powerhouse

Lauki delivers essential vitamins like C, B, K, A and E, and minerals like iron, folate and manganese. Not many people know how brilliant a source of vitamin C this understated food is: 250 gm of lauki delivers 25 mg of vitamin C, which meets half our daily requirement. Vitamin C helps us make collagen, a protein that is essential for tissue strength and also prevents wrinkles and the premature ageing of the skin.

The B vitamins also help delay greying of hair, and zinc keeps cold and flu away and our nerves strong.

## Easy on the Stomach

Lauki is very easy to digest, so it is a perfect food for summer months when our digestive system does not work at its optimum. The soluble and insoluble fibre it delivers keeps our digestion humming, and constipation, piles and flatulence away.

## A Weight Loss Tool

Lauki is a brilliant weight loss food. Even 100 gm of the vegetable delivers just 15 calories (YES!). Also, the nutrients and fibre in it help keep us satisfied and thus, keep the cravings away. Vitamin K keeps our metabolism robust.

> **Did You Know?**
> According to Ayurveda, lauki is our liver's best friend, an organ that needs a lot of help in today's highly toxic times. It helps cut liver inflammation actively.

## Beat the Blues

Thanks to the good amount of choline, a kind of neurotransmitter that improves the functions of the brain and helps prevent stress, depression and other mental disorders, lauki has a sedative effect on us. It actually calms and relaxes us. So, to chase away those blues, maybe along with meditation, all you need is a bowl of lauki for lunch.

## Easy Tips to Eat Bottle Gourds

Lauki has a neutral flavour and is easy to cook. It can be transformed into spectacular dishes with a play of masalas.

Move beyond just lauki subzi and lauki koftas, and try to experiment a bit. Try stuffing it with boiled potatoes and then dousing it in a thick gravy; or simply blanch it, stuff with cottage cheese and bake it. Chana dal with ghiya is a perennial favourite, so is a cool lauki raita. It lends itself well to sweet dishes too—lauki barfi and halwa are extremely popular.

## Juice It!

The easiest way to increase the consumption of lauki is to juice it. This is good for everyone, especially diabetics, as it stabilizes the blood sugar level and maintains the blood pressure.

To make it, you can just peel the lauki, cut it into pieces, and blend it. Add black pepper, salt and mint leaves. Add 1 tsp of ginger paste to the juice. Finally, squeeze some lemon juice in. Have it quickly as it oxidizes quite fast.

Lauki juice helps lower the blood cholesterol level, and as it is extremely alkalizing and an effective diuretic, it also helps treat urinary tract infections and lower uric acid level. The best time to have it is in the morning to neutralize the acids in the stomach and correct hormonal imbalances.

And this one will surprise you! If you exercise, then post your workout, a glass of this juice, thanks to the natural sugars it delivers, can help restore both your glucose levels and electrolyte balance. For quick muscle recovery, just grate in some ginger to the mix.

These are enough reasons to have lauki twice or thrice a week when in season, right?

**At a Glance**

The benefits of eating lauki include,

- Natural cooling of the body
- Boosting the mood
- Quick muscle recovery
- Getting lots of vitamin C
- Cleaning the digestive tract
- Lowering blood pressure

**Fun Fact**

Lauki comes in all sizes—from 4 inches to 40 inches in length, and 2 inches to 12 inches in diameter.

Chapter 7

# CARROT

## Why Eating Carrots Is a Very Clever Idea

How many times do you have gajar ka halwa when carrots are in season?

If you don't, then this chapter is going to make you drool and make you rush hotfoot to your nearest vegetables market to buy carrots, a root vegetable packed with nutrition and yet highly underrated, which can be traced back to about 5,000 years through historical documents and paintings. In fact, it is so good for us that in ancient times, it was grown as medicine, not food.

There's so much to love about carrots–their crunchy texture, sweet taste, easy availability and the fact that they are inexpensive. Still, they are not eaten as much as they should be when in season.

## Nutrient Load

Low in calories (150 gm, that is, 2 large carrots deliver just 60 calories), carrots are a good source of fibre (4 gm) and multiple nutrients like vitamins A, C and K, as well as pantothenic acid (B5), folate (B9), potassium, iron, copper and manganese.

**Did You Know?**
Carrots don't actually contain vitamin A, but they're an excellent source of beta-carotene, the antioxidant carotenoid that gets converted to vitamin A in the body.

## The Car(r)otene Queen

Carotene helps boost our immunity and eye health. Carrots are loaded with carotenoids, lutein and zeaxanthin, that help reduce the risk of age-related deterioration of the retina.

The diabetes preventive effects of carotenoids, besides their link to reduced risks of several cancers, notably lung and prostate cancer, are also becoming clear now. And although carrots are considered a sweet vegetable (and thus shunned by many), the carotenoids in them help regulate the amount of insulin and glucose being metabolized in the body, and so they actually actively help lower blood sugar and help diabetics stay healthy. They should, of course, be eaten in moderation (2 small carrots a day is good) as they do contain more sugar compared to other vegetables (besides beet).

## A Boon for Your Bones

The beta-carotene present in carrots helps keep the bones healthy. The vitamin C and calcium in carrots help the bones too.

## Detox and De-stress

Carotenoids present in carrots are a fat-soluble vitamin, so they stimulate bile in the liver to flow and hasten the removal of toxins. Another benefit of carrots is that they are a good source of the difficult-to-find vitamin B8 (also known as inositol), which is known for its stress- and anxiety-busting properties, and for boosting our mental health and cognitive function. Carrots are also rich in luteolin, which helps keep your memory buzzing and also to cut brain inflammation. Beta-carotene also helps keep our memory in good shape by protecting the central nervous system.

### Save Your Heart

Carrots, because of their high soluble fibre content, largely pectin, have been found to help cut down cholesterol in the body. As they are a rich source of potassium, which is a vasodilator, they help relax tension in the blood vessels and arteries and boost blood flow and circulation. Coumarin, a natural compound found in carrots, also helps keep blood pressure tamed and hypertension away, besides preventing asthma and osteoporosis.

### Easy Tips to Eat Carrots

With carrots, the idea is to include them in both raw and cooked form in the diet, as both kinds deliver different benefits. When cooked, there is indeed some loss of minerals and water-soluble vitamins, but the availability of antioxidants, particularly beta-carotene absorption, is maximized. Cook carrots with a small amount of fat, as this antioxidant becomes more accessible to the body when its tough cell walls are slightly broken down.

So, besides gajar halwa, which you must eat, and kanji, which is a brilliant probiotic drink, you can simply roast them, or sauté them in olive oil, or steam and puree them to make a rich, creamy soup. Add shredded carrots and chopped carrot greens to salads or combine shredded carrots, beets and apples, and eat as a salad.

Like it spicy? Bake carrot sticks, olive oil, honey, paprika, salt and pepper in a preheated oven at 400°F for 20 minutes; turn and bake further for 10 minutes. Or make spiced carrot sticks by soaking them in hot water with some cayenne, coriander (dhania) seeds and salt. Allow to cool, drain and serve.

Try this quick recipe too: Slice carrots ¼-inch thick and steam/microwave for 5 minutes. Coat with 1 tbsp maple syrup (or honey) and 1 tbsp mustard while the carrots are hot. Dig in. It's a fancy, delicious, and less-than-100-calorie snack that satisfies the sweet tooth as well.

### At a Glance

The benefits of eating carrots include,

- Preventing diabetes
- Netting greater bone mass
- Protecting the central nervous system against ageing
- Detoxifying and de-stressing
- Saving your heart

### Fun Fact
We think of carrots as orange and red, but they can also be white, yellow and purple.

Chapter 8

# CASHEW

### Eat Cashews Minus Any Guilt

Take a guess: Which nut gets rapped the most?

Cashew nuts, of course. They have been on the receiving end of bad press for, well, forever. This is thanks to the all-prevailing myth that they raise cholesterol, and also maybe because they are delicious. And something so tasty cannot really be good for us, right?

Wrong, actually.

I love to eat this nut, without any guilt. In fact, I carry them around in my bag as a saviour for the times when I have mild hunger pangs. This comma-shaped kernel does not make your waist wider and your life shorter. In fact, regular consumption of cashew nuts actually helps boost our health by leading to a drop in systolic blood pressure and increasing the good cholesterol, HDL. These nuts also do not have any negative influence on body weight, glucose or bad cholesterol, LDL.

So how does this happen? It's actually the good-fat content of cashews, the monounsaturated fatty acids (MUFA), which help. We traditionally follow diets that are deficient in MUFA, and that is bad news for our heart health. Cashews, with their MUFA content, actually help fill this gap. Another benefit is that they have a lower amount of fat (13 gm per ounce) compared to other nuts.

Secondly, most of the saturated fat in cashews is stearic

acid, which does not affect our blood lipids negatively.

This is why the common scare about cashews messing our cholesterol levels is unfounded. For starters, they have absolutely no cholesterol content in them; rather they actually help cut down bad cholesterol level in the body, while jacking up the good cholesterol.

## Nutrient-filled Nut

Cashew nuts deliver antioxidants and plant sterols and are loaded with proanthocyanidins (flavanols) that stop cancer cells from multiplying and are also loaded with hard-to-find micronutrients like vitamins E, K and B6, and minerals like copper, phosphorus, zinc, magnesium, iron and selenium.

Phosphorus is essential for teeth and bones, selenium protects against cancer, zinc strengthens the immune system and thyroid glands, and copper helps absorb iron better and eliminate free radicals from the body. Copper is also essential for healthy hair as it is needed for the production of the skin and hair pigment called melanin. Magnesium boosts the immune system, keeps the bones strong and helps maintain blood pressure.

Cashews actually are a good package as the good fats in them help the body absorb the fat-soluble vitamins A, D, E and K, and produce essential fatty acids.

### Did You Know?
Cashews contain a powerful antioxidant pigment called zeaxanthin, which forms a protective layer over our retina and saves it from the harmful effects of ultraviolet rays, keeping our eyes healthy.

### Finally...

There is no danger of weight gain despite cashews being high in calories—an ounce delivers 160 calories and about 5 gm of protein—and they are comparatively low in fibre as compared to other nuts, as they are a highly satieting food. A moderate intake of unsalted nuts and those not roasted in unhealthy oils or ghee is actually good for us.

### Easy Tips to Eat Cashews

Now that you know that when you munch on cashews, they are doing you lots of good, go on, include them in your diet without any fear. Munch on them, add to dishes like poha, dalia and upma, and use liberally in cakes and muffins. In fact, I say celebrate cashews without any worries.

### At a Glance

The benefits of eating cashews include,

- Cutting down bad cholesterol
- Loading up on antioxidants
- Staying satiated for long
- Brain development
- Proper blood clotting

#### Fun Fact
In Goa, the juice extracted from cashews is fermented and made into a drink called feni or fenny, which has about 40-42 per cent alcohol.

Mini Chapter II

## BEAT THE BLOAT

**Fixit Tip 15:** In order to beat water retention, get enough magnesium in your diet. Depend on nuts (especially almonds), legumes, wheat, green vegetables, potatoes, apples, jamun, phalsa, mangoes, amla, guavas and bananas.

**Fixit Tip 16:** Eat one food with diuretic properties everyday: celery, lettuce, carrot, onion, asparagus, tomato or cucumber.

**Fixit Tip 17:** It makes absolute sense to go back to that age-old practice of adding coriander leaves over veggies; these greens are natural diuretics, and also aid in digestion.

**Fixit Tip 18:** Parsley tea is an effective solution for bloating (diuretic). Brew 2 tsp dried leaves per cup of boiling water and steep for 10 minutes. Drink up to three cups a day.

**Fixit Tip 19:** An excellent source of potassium and fibre, figs are a good source of vitamin B6 too, which helps prevent water retention.

**Fixit Tip 20:** Boil fennel seeds (saunf) in water, and let it cool. Drinking this helps flush out excess fluids from the body and purge out toxins.

Chapter 9

# CAULIFLOWER

## Let Us Talk about Cauliflower

We have never taken cauliflower (gobhi) seriously, and by 'we', I mean chefs, nutrition experts, or even home cooks. You do not see it being hyped in the media because no one writes about it (unlike, say a broccoli, which is considered 'cool'). This is possibly because it is so easily accessible (every vegetable vendor has it), inexpensive, and has always been cooked in our homes, almost by rotation a couple of times a week at least. My mom feels it pairs well with every dal, and thinks it is a perfect addition to the menu whenever you need to add another veggie to the table if you want to make the meal more elaborate or if someone is coming over for dinner.

When a vegetable is so giving and dependable like the cauliflower is, even if it doesn't ask for it and doesn't have serious backers, it still needs to be talked about. The simple, humble aloo gobhi spiced with turmeric (haldi) and cumin (jeera), which you have been eating from childhood, has been doing you a lot of good. You need to know this so that, if cauliflower isn't being made much in your home currently, this is a reminder that it should.

## A Bonafide Weight Loss Food

For starters, this is an extremely low-calorie vegetable that delivers a bundle of fibre too. One cup of cauliflower or about 120 gm gives you just 25 calories and a whopping 3 gm of fibre. This makes it a brilliant food for keeping our digestive system happy, and can work as a low-calorie substitute for many high-calorie foods, such as rice and flour. This is probably why the keto dieters have embraced this vegetable so fervently. Don't blame them: 1 cup of cauliflower delivers 5 gm of carbs compared to 1 cup of rice, which contains 45 gm of carbs (9 times more!).

## Loaded with Nutrients

It contains some of almost every vitamin and mineral that you need, being an excellent source of vitamins C, K and B, and minerals like potassium, manganese, magnesium, phosphorus.

## Cuts Cancer and Heart Disease

The antioxidants glucosinolates and isothiocyanates in cauliflower help slow the growth of cancer cells. These are especially protective against colon, lung, breast and prostate cancer. Cauliflowers also deliver another antioxidant called sulforaphane, which can even destroy cells that are already damaged by cancer. They keep the heart in the pink of health by taming our blood pressure and keeping the arteries healthy. Also, the vitamin C in cauliflower works as an antioxidant and anti-inflammatory agent and helps reduce the risk of heart disease and cancer.

### Did You Know?
Cauliflower also has the ability to bind together with bile acids and help regulate blood cholesterol levels.

### The Choline Advantage

Cauliflower delivers one of the rare nutrients found in foods, choline, which our body needs for the brain and nervous system to function properly. Choline delivers another bonus: it helps prevent cholesterol from accumulating in the liver and thus reduces the risk of liver and heart diseases, dementia and Alzheimer's.

### Easy Tips to Eat Cauliflowers

Getting a little experimental in the kitchen always helps. Be it with ingredients, seasonings, or even just the way we cut the veggies or cook them. With cauliflower being considered bland and boring by many, experimentation really helps. The best way to get all the health benefits of this vegetable is to sauté and eat it (instead of boiling or steaming). Cooking may lead to loss of some water-soluble nutrients but it also increases the availability of other nutrients like carotenoids, lutein and zeaxanthin (great for our eye health). So make cauliflower rice, add it to soups, or try making a pizza base or hummus with it.

And next time instead of mashed potatoes, try cauliflower mash—it is healthier and even more delicious. Just discard the core, separate the florets and steam them till tender. Add a little milk, butter, sour cream, seasoning (salt and pepper) to taste, and mash with a masher.

### At a Glance

The benefits of eating cauliflower include,

- Strengthening your nerves
- Boosting digestive health
- Losing weight

- Cutting cholesterol
- Reducing cancer and heart disease risk

**Fun Fact**

The most common cauliflowers are those in a creamy white hue, but this vegetable actually comes in a variety of bright colours like purple and orange, which are delicious and healthy too.

Chapter 10

# CHICKPEA

### Catch 'em Chickpeas

Chickpeas, also known as garbanzo beans, are the big daddy of legumes. Dating back about 7,500 years, these are eaten extensively across the world. And for good reason!

The two kinds of chickpeas—desi (Bengal gram or kala chana) and kabuli (safed chana) are nutrition powerhouses: ½ cup cooked chickpeas (80 gm) will give about 130 calories, 7 gm protein (a great protein source for vegetarians), 6.5 gm fibre, 2.5 mg hard-to-find zinc and multiple other vitamins and minerals.

### Hunger Control

You can stay full for long with these super-healthy legumes as they are loaded with fibre, which helps fill you up with less; in fact, it has been noticed that the urge to snack is lower after eating chickpeas. Its fibre content also lowers cholesterol and triglycerides in the body, making it extremely heart healthy. Here, desi chickpeas score better than kabulis, as they have higher fibre and thus a very low glycemic index, making them great for diabetics too.

### Antioxidants Ahoy!

Packed with antioxidants—vitamins C and E, and beta-carotene—chickpeas are rich in coveted phytonutrients, and have loads of manganese too (1 cup gives 40 mg, almost half our daily requirement). Here too, the desi variety with its thicker seed coat, stores a greater concentration.

## A Woman's Friend

The phytoestrogens in chickpeas help protect against osteoporosis and lower the risk of breast cancer. How it works is this—when we eat chickpeas, its fibre gets fermented in the gut to form butyrate, a short-chain fatty acid. Butyrate helps induce apoptosis (self-destruction) of cancerous cells. Impressive, isn't it?

### Did You Know?
All you insomniacs out there, please note that as chickpeas are a high-tryptophan food, they can help calm your mind and lull you to deep sleep too.

## Easy Tips to Eat Chickpeas

Target eating half a cup of cooked chickpeas (alternating between both types) thrice a week, at least. Make a nice, spicy chickpea curry and pair it with rice. After all, who doesn't like chhole chawal? However, get a little experimental too (they are very versatile, try them). Add them to salads and soups, roast them (drizzle olive oil, roast at 400°F for 30–40 minutes, and add salt), or try making falafel and hummus (look up Part III of the book for the recipe).

Also try sprouted chickpeas (their nutrients skyrocket this way). Fancy a bowl meal? Mix cooked dalia, boiled chickpeas, steamed and shredded carrots and cabbage (patta gobhi), and raw moong dal sprouts, and top with green chutney or salsa.

## At a Glance

The benefits of eating chickpeas include,
- Staying full for long
- Scoring multiple antioxidants
- Gaining protection against osteoporosis
- Lowering the risk of breast cancer
- Sleeping better

### Fun Fact

In the Philippines, chickpeas preserved in syrup are eaten as dessert. Good idea, I say!

Chapter 11

# CORN

**Corn Makes Life Crunchier and Better**

So, what's your corn-on-the-cob (bhutta) memory? Most people have one dating back to childhood. It could be the one they had at a hill station, with the rain for company; or the one they had with their grandpa in the village. Actually, there are no excuses to not pick a crisp cob smeared with lots of lemon and masala, and bite into it when it is in season. It's a better bet than any fried snack and, trust me, more satisfying too.

**Nutrition Load**

Corn, called maize in most countries (it comes from the Spanish word 'maíz'), might be slightly steep in calories (250 gm gives about 215 calories) but an average bhutta should be about half of that, which is not a bad deal. Also, it has a mere 2 per cent fat content and no cholesterol. Being highly calorific, it actually proves to be a boon for those who are looking to gain weight.

These little yellow kernels pack a protein punch (8 gm), but as the amino acids—lysine and isoleucine—are missing, it makes sense to eat it paired with cheese, tofu, nuts, or cooked lentils to ensure you get complete protein.

## Eye and Heart Tonic

Corn is loaded with lutein, zeaxanthin and carotenoids, which help keep our eyes healthy and functioning at their best. Lutein also prevents the build-up of fatty deposits in arteries (a common cause for heart attacks). Corn also has phenols (phytochemicals) that help keep hypertension away.

> **Did You Know?**
> Corn is great for your skin health as the antioxidants, vitamin C and lycopene, that it delivers help boost the production of collagen and also prevent skin damage from ultraviolet-generated free radicals.

## The B Advantage

Corn is loaded with vitamin B. It delivers lots of thiamin, which is a boon for our brain's health; niacin, which brings bad cholesterol levels down; folic acid, which is important for the production of red blood cells; and pantothenic acid (B5), which helps metabolize carbohydrates, proteins and lipids properly in the body. Folic acid is great for our heart too as it keeps the level of homocysteine down in the body (elevation of which is linked to a higher heart disease risk). The important thing about B vitamins is that they are water soluble, so they're not stored in the body. This means that we need to get them from our diet regularly. It makes a good case for a bhutta a day, doesn't it?

## Loads of Minerals too

Corn delivers multiple minerals too: phosphorous, magnesium, manganese, zinc, iron and copper, and trace mineral selenium (difficult to find otherwise), which helps prevent mental decline.

## Keeps Blood Sugar Stable

Worried about corn being high on carbs? Don't be, because corn is associated with better blood sugar control. That's probably because it is packed with both fibre and protein, and both ensure a stable passage of food through our digestive tract (helps avoid too rapid or too slow a digestion of food). This prevents sudden spikes or drops in blood sugar. Another payoff is the higher satiety that it provides. In fact, phytochemicals found in corn can regulate the absorption and release of insulin in the body, which can reduce the chance of spikes and drops for diabetics.

## Your Gut's Friend

A whopping 5 gm fibre is delivered by 250 gm corn, which, besides giving us plenty of chewing satisfaction, keeps our digestion humming along nicely and constipation away too. That's great for the monsoon time (when corn is usually in season too) as our digestion gets a little sluggish during that time. Corn does so much good for our gut, thanks to its high ratio of insoluble-to-soluble fibre. The soluble fibre that corn has, actually forms short-chain fatty acids (SCFAs) in the intestines, which, besides being great for our gut, also helps keep colon cancer away.

## Easy Tips to Eat Corn

Besides corn on the cob that can be relished in a roasted or steamed form, try corn bhel, grilled corn sandwiches, corn patties, corn samosas and baked corn.

Feeling adventurous? Try making corn biryani, or

sprinkle some on your pizza. You could, of course, just steam corn kernels in a tangy olive oil-salt-pepper-herbs dressing and enjoy.

## At a Glance

The benefits of eating corn include,

- Strengthening your gut
- Protecting your skin from ultraviolet rays
- Boosting your eyesight
- Getting a protein punch
- Preventing mental decline
- Keeping blood sugar stable
- Gaining a healthy weight

### Fun Fact
An ear or cob of corn is actually part of the flower, and each kernel is a seed. Also, a cob always has an even number of rows.

Chapter 12

# CUSTARD APPLE

### Beat Pollution with Custard Apple

Living with pollution today is a huge problem. Hardly anyone is able to escape from it, especially if you live in a large city. It's difficult to ignore the breaths of toxic air that we take in every second, and no solution seems to be in sight. However, there is actually one simple solution that can help. Consuming the elusive vitamin B6, pyridoxin, can help reduce the bronchial (tubes that go to the lungs) inflammation that is caused by the toxic air we breathe. Not many know that the understated custard apple, known as sharifa or sitaphal in Hindi, is loaded with it. That is why eating it can actually help keep you safer by cleaning your lungs. It also helps prevent asthmatic attacks.

### It Is Not Highly Calorific

Custard apples are not eaten much, as most people believe that they're high in calories (just because they're so sweet). That is not true. 100 gm of custard apple gives close to 100 calories only, which is nothing compared to the goodness that comes packed in this fruit. In fact, because it is so sweet, it is a perfect replacement for empty high-calorie desserts. It is also an effective fatigue buster and energy-giving food. What I personally love about it (besides its sweet taste) is that you just cannot eat it really fast (because of so many seeds) and have to savour it slowly. So you can never have too much of it.

## Nutrient Dense

It is sodium- and cholesterol-free and is an excellent source of fibre, vitamins B6 (pyridoxine) and C, potassium, manganese and copper. It also delivers some other B vitamins—B1 and B2—as well as zinc, magnesium and iron.

## A (Custard) Apple a Day

Besides being great for our lungs, B6 keeps our nervous system in good health too. It helps in the production of neurotransmitters, which are important for our brain's functioning and to prevent cognitive decline.

B6 is also involved in the production of haemoglobin, whose deficiency leads to anaemia, fatigue and low energy. A custard apple a day can help keep anaemia away.

It also makes sitaphal a 'happy fruit' as it is needed to produce the hormones serotonin, which helps regulate mood; norepinephrine, which is essential to cope with stress; and melatonin, which helps us sleep better.

## Your Skin's Friend

Vitamin A in custard apple works as an anti-ageing and moisturizing agent, and helps keep our eyesight sharp. Custard apple also decreases the clustering of melanin granules, which reduces brown spots and pigmentation on the skin.

## The Antioxidant Quota

Custard apple also has loads of the antioxidant vitamin C, which protects us from free radicals, the harbingers of most lifestyle diseases. Vitamin C is also anti-inflammatory and immune boosting. Antioxidants asimicin and bullatacin found in it have shown anti-cancer properties.

> **Did You Know?**
> Custard apple delivers a decent amount of calcium too, which is vital for bone health.

## The Fibre Advantage

Custard apple also contains a significant amount of fibre (2.4 gm per 100 gm), which protects the colon membrane and helps flush out the toxins from the intestine, aiding in proper functioning of the bowels. A lot of people think that diabetics should avoid this fruit as it is sweet, but that is a myth as the fibre in custard apple actually slows down the absorption of sugar in the body. In fact, moderate amounts of it might actually benefit diabetics as it leads to the stimulation of insulin production and increases the uptake of glucose by muscles, which helps stabilize blood sugar levels. The vitamin C and magnesium in it also help in stimulating the insulin in the body and thus, in glucose regulation.

## There's More!

Custard apple delivers high potassium, which helps keep our blood pressure tamed and fights muscle weakness; the magnesium present in it protects our heart. The fruit also contains compounds like acetogenin and alkaloids, which reduce the risk of cancer and renal failure.

## Easy Tips to Eat Custard Apples

The easiest way to eat custard apples is to just cut it in half or pull apart with your hands and use a spoon to scoop out the flesh. Try adding a little lime juice; it adds a lovely flavour. Like most tropical fruits, chilling actually dulls the flavour, so it should be enjoyed at room temperature. You can use the flesh raw in fruit salads, ice creams, milk shakes and yoghurt smoothies too. Also, have you ever tried sitaphal phirni? You'll never go back to regular phirni once you do. My friend's mother used to make sitaphal kalakand as well, which was delicious. See if you can source the recipe from somewhere!

**At a Glance**

The benefits of eating custard apple include,

- Boosting brain health
- Keeping your lungs clean
- Beating anaemia
- Protecting the heart
- Strengthening the bones

### Fun Fact
Native to South America and the West Indies, custard apple is called 'Buddha Head fruit' in Taiwan.

Mini Chapter III

## DISEASE BUSTERS

**Fixit Tip 21:** Eating 5–6 gm (1 tsp) of fennel seeds every day helps in improving the functioning of the liver.

**Fixit Tip 22:** Chew 5–9 holy basil (tulsi) leaves every morning. Holy basil has a high level of potassium, magnesium and vitamin C, which help in regulating your blood pressure. It is a mood stabilizer too.

**Fixit Tip 23:** To prevent diabetes, take 2 tsp powdered fenugreek (methi) seeds every morning with a spoonful of honey. Or soak fenugreek seeds overnight in a cup of water, drink the water the next morning and chew the seeds. It helps decrease insulin response.

**Fixit Tip 24:** Compounds found in bitter gourds (karela) activate an enzyme known as adenosine 5' monophosphate-activated protein kinase, or AMPK, which helps to regulate glucose metabolism. This helps prevent diabetes and also helps diabetics use the insulin they produce more effectively.

**Fixit Tip 25:** Turnips (shalgam) are loaded with potassium, which helps bring blood pressure down. With just around 30 calories per 100 gm, they are a lower-calorie choice than the same amount of another high-potassium food, let's say, boiled potatoes (almost 80 calories).

**Fixit Tip 26:** Turnip greens contain about twice the calcium content as compared to mustard greens and are also packed with glucosinolates (phytonutrients) that help prevent cancer.

**Fixit Tip 27:** Pistachios aren't bad for us. They, in fact, are especially rich in vitamin B6, which is important for keeping hormones balanced and healthy.

**Fixit Tip 28:** Do you have anaemia? Focus on tamarind (imli). It has both iron and vitamin C, so it is a good source of better-absorbed iron for vegetarians.

**Fixit Tip 29:** Green bananas (also known as plantains), besides having bone-strengthening fructooligosaccharides (like ripe bananas), also offer short-chain fatty acids, making them twice as effective at strengthening our bones.

Try this salad: Boil a plantain for 10 minutes and then slice it; mix with a sliced carrot, cucumber, celery and lettuce; sprinkle peanuts and drizzle a dressing of your choice.

Or just chop a plantain, coat the slices with some oil and bake. Then have with homemade spicy tomato sauce.

**Fixit Tip 30:** Mineral silicon, though lesser-known compared to calcium and magnesium, is extremely important for bone health and for the healthy formation of connective tissue. French beans are loaded with it.

**Fixit Tip 31:** You really are (as bright as) what you eat. Tyrosine, an amino acid found in spinach, cottage cheese (paneer) and soya, is linked to enhanced reflexes and intellectual capabilities. Now that's an easy and inexpensive way of boosting our brainpower, wouldn't your agree?

**Fixit Tip 32:** Grapes have a lot of boron, which is necessary for good bone health and protects against osteoporosis.

**Fixit Tip 33:** Pomegranate has a miracle antioxidant compound punicalagin (a polyphenol), which can prevent Alzheimer's and even slow its onset and progression. Chomp on it, juice it, or add to couscous, raita and salads.

**Fixit Tip 34:** If tomato is not your best friend already, please remedy that right away! Lycopene, which tomato is loaded with, is linked to reduction of heart diseases. In fact, lycopene is ten times more powerful than vitamin E and its benefit gets enhanced when it is consumed cooked, like in purees and chutneys.

**Fixit Tip 35:** Eat at least one of these everyday—peanuts, cashews or pumpkin seeds—to get enough zinc. Low zinc levels can predispose a person to Alzheimer's disease.

**Fixit Tip 36:** Combining unsaturated fats with nitrite-rich vegetables, for example, nuts with spinach or carrots, can protect you from hypertension. So, eat this combination regularly.

**Fixit Tip 37:** Strawberries are loaded with anthocyanins (flavonoids), which lower blood pressure, make blood vessels more elastic and help prevent hypertension.

**Fixit Tip 38:** Eating sliced raw onions with your meals will do a lot of good for your heart. Sulphur in onion acts as a natural blood thinner and prevents blood platelets from aggregating, and the antioxidant quercetin helps prevent plaque build-up in the arteries. Both quercetin and sulphur also help keep our immunity buffed up.

**Fixit Tip 39:** The seeds in grapes contain a substance called pyenogenols, which fights arthritis, stress and allergies.

**Fixit Tip 40:** Okra's (bhindi) sliminess makes it hard for some people to love it, but it's also what makes it so good for you. It is loaded with soluble fibre (like the fibre found in oats). Also, okra's mucilage helps lower blood cholesterol levels tremendously.

**Fixit Tip 41:** Tomatoes are a very good source of chromium, which helps to regulate blood sugar.

**Fixit Tip 42:** Apricot (kubaani) is an excellent remedy for anaemia because of its high iron content. Also, the small but essential amount of copper in the fruit makes iron available to the body.

Chapter 13

# DATE

### Plan a Date with a Date

Dates (khajoor) are not just to break the Ramadan fast; they are perfect otherwise too. If you ask me, dates are actually a saviour. Particularly for those who have a sweet tooth, and even for those who need to cut down on their sugar and fat intake because of a health issue, as dates are a fat-free food, making them a delicious alternative to high-fat desserts. Even otherwise, unlike sugar, they are actually good for us.

They are a favourite for breaking the fast during the Ramadan month as they instantly replenish energy and revitalize a tired body. They are also hugely treasured by those who do intermittent fasting. But that aside, there are lots of other reasons why they are perfect.

### Fasting Panacea

First, they are easy to digest so they don't overwhelm the stomach after a long fasting period. In fact, they activate digestive secretions and prepare our stomach for more food. They also feed our brain cells and nerves immediately and instantly, which is much-needed after a long period of scarcity. They help prevent constipation that could result due to low-fibre intake during days of intermittent eating.

### Energy Boosters

They are big energy boosters and therefore, perfect for the summer months when fatigue is rampant. Actually, that's precisely also why they have been a favourite of nomads in deserts. Since ancient times, they have been providing life-sustaining nutrition in places of sparse vegetation. Today, this attribute makes them a good pre- and post-workout snack for all fitness enthusiasts.

Tip: To help beat that rundown feeling, take 3–4 pieces of dates and boil them with one glass of milk or water. Eat the dates and drink the milk or water. It will give you instant energy, and hydrate you effectively too. This combination (milk and dates) is also known for its ability to maintain a healthy nervous system and heart.

### Better than Sugar

In spite of being high in sugar (fructose) and glycemic index (which can increase blood sugar levels significantly), dates are still a good alternative for sugar. That's because, unlike sugar, which delivers only empty calories, dates deliver a stockpile of nutrients too—about 30 gm (4 dates) provides around 90 calories, 1 gm protein, 2.3 gm fibre, 13 mg calcium, and multiple other nutrients.

### Nutrition Overload

Dates deliver a lot of B vitamins, particularly B6, which is known to boost brain performance and better test scores. They also deliver vitamin K, which is brilliant for our bones, and their vitamin A content helps keep our vision sharp, safeguards against night blindness and keeps our skin happy. They also have zeaxanthin, which protects against age-related vision loss.

## Mineral Master

This tiny food is, in fact, known as a mineral master, because it contains a small amount of almost every essential mineral, like calcium, magnesium and manganese, which are important for calcium absorption and for producing sex hormones; zinc, which protects from cold and flu and boosts immunity; copper, which helps in the production of red blood cells and helps the brain function properly; iron to keep anaemia away; and selenium, potassium and more. It also has fluorine, which prevents cavities. You can easily substitute dates for sugar without guilt, and score a stockpile of nutrients in the bargain.

## Heart-friendly

Free of saturated fat, trans fat, sodium and cholesterol, they are a heart-friendly food, and are known to lower bad cholesterol (LDL) in the body. Also, their potassium content helps control heart rate, and keeps blood pressure regulated. As they are high in potassium and low in sodium, they work wonders for our nervous system too.

## Antioxidant Activity

Dates are not just a sweet bite, they also contain antioxidants called polyphenols, which help to purge out toxins (free radicals) from the body and help detox it. They also cut inflammation in the body and protect us from inflammatory disorders.

> **Did You Know?**
> Eating dates soaked overnight is a proven remedy for hangovers too, and they also help detoxify the body.

### There's More!

Dates are known to increase sexual stamina. Their high levels of estradiol and flavonoid components increase sperm count and motility. That's why they have been used as an aphrodisiac since ages.

### Brilliant Digester

Dates are loaded with fibre, both soluble and insoluble, which help regulate blood sugar, keep us satiated, lower blood cholesterol and keep our gastrointestinal tract happy. They promote friendly bacteria in the intestines, and the fibre in them keeps constipation at bay. If your stomach has been playing up, then too dates help, as they are a natural laxative.

### Easy Tips to Eat Dates

Eating 3–4 dates a day is a good idea. Soak and have them in the morning, or add them to shakes and sprinkle on puddings, kheer, custard, oats and muesli.

Stuffed dates are interesting too. Stuff them with almonds, pecans, cream cheese, or pistachios for a snack or finger food.

### At a Glance

The benefits of eating dates include,

- Improving the complexion
- Improving vision
- Lowering cholesterol
- Strengthening the gut
- Getting energized

## Fun Fact
Bedouin tribes of the Middle East, who eat lots of dates every day, have one of the lowest rates of cancer in the world.

Chapter 14

# EGGPLANT

## Learn to Love the Eggplant

Eggplant (also called baingan, brinjal and aubergine) is not a popular food, probably because of its bland looks and slightly bitter taste. That's a pity because it has everything going for it.

## 'Stay Thin' Panacea

Eggplant is about 95 per cent water, so it is a perfect 'stay thin' food. It is ridiculously low in calories (25 calories per 100 gm) and loaded with fibre (3 gm), so you can eat a lot of it and still not gain weight at all. It is also packed with a bunch of B vitamins (especially B6), choline, folate, pantothenic acid, riboflavin, niacin and thiamine, all of which help keep our metabolism running, a prerequisite for staying thin.

## The Amazing Antioxidants

Eggplants deliver a lot of antioxidants, particularly chlorogenic acid, a wonder pigment that works on four fronts: fights free radicals and many viruses, lowers LDL (bad cholesterol), and provides protection against cancer. For this compound alone, it makes sense to eat more of this spongy vegetable. They are loaded with another antioxidant, anthocyanin, which is a proven cancer slayer, anti-ageing panacea, inflammation cutter, and is heart protective too.

## Your Heart's Friend

Besides being weighing scale-friendly, there are a lot of other reasons to plate this food more often. Anthocyanins present in eggplant help protect our heart. It is also a high potassium and low-sodium food, which again is good news for our heart. The chlorogenic acid in it helps lower LDL levels. Both anthocyanins and chlorogenic acid are effective cancer slayers too.

### Did You Know?
Eggplant helps prevent diabetes, thanks to its high-fibre and low soluble carbohydrate content.

## Gut-friendly

Eggplant is a perfect antidote to the junk food we eat so much these days. Junk food makes our gut acidic, which is a harbinger of diseases, and eggplant helps moderate the pH of our gut, makes our gastro system alkaline and keeps us healthy. Also, it is a natural laxative, thanks to the amount of fibre in it that keeps our bowels working fine, and prevents constipation.

## Don't Throw Away the Skin

An eggplant's skin is full of fibre, potassium, magnesium and antioxidants. The phenols in it are potent free radical scavengers, which help keep myriad lifestyle diseases away! Nasunin, an anthocyanin found within its skin, is known to boost the brain, protect it from free radical damage and improve memory.

## Easy Tips to Eat Eggplants

It is very easy to put more of this versatile food on your plate. It can be roasted, grilled, steamed, or sautéed. You can just stick to the tried-and-tested age-old Indian recipes like baingan ka bharta, stuffed brinjal, or a baingan curry with cauliflower and tomatoes. I totally dig the regular aloo-baingan subzi made at home, and also always keep homemade baba ganoush handy (purée roasted eggplant, garlic, tahini, lemon juice and olive oil).

Try not to fry them, because they have a tendency to soak up a lot of oil. And if you don't quite like their slightly bitter taste, then just cut them, sprinkle some salt on them, let them rest for a bit, then squeeze and rinse with water once.

Also try this: Grill eggplant slices tossed with a bit of oil, salt and pepper for 5 minutes, flipping once. Place atop a slice of bread grilled with cheese, garlic and herbs, and dig in.

## At a Glance

The benefits of eating eggplant include,

- Losing weight
- Scoring amazing antioxidants
- Improving your memory
- Preventing diabetes
- Countering the ill effects of the junk food you eat

### Fun Fact
Sixteenth-century Europeans called eggplant 'mad apple' as they thought eating it will make them mad (because it belongs to the toxic nightshade family of plants).

Chapter 15

# POHA

### India's Own Fast Food

Whenever I go to Krishna's own land, Barsana, near Mathura in Uttar Pradesh, I always eat poha (beaten rice, flattened rice, rice flakes, atkulu or aval) to the heart's content. I am a huge poha fan–have always been–and somehow eating it there has its own charm. After all, who has not grown up hearing the story about Sudama's gift of poha to his childhood friend Krishna and how much the Lord loved it?

I love the fact that I have something in common with Krishna: Poha was his favourite food too! Another reason why I totally dig this humble food is because of how healthy and nutritious this simple, underrated dish is!

I eat it a couple of times every week for breakfast (often as a light lunch too) but unfortunately, I don't see too many people doing that anymore and that is a pity.

### Easily Digestible

Do you know why it is considered an excellent weaning food, and a home remedy for treating an upset tummy or fever? That is because it is an easily digestible food, and everyone from infants to elderly people can handle it. Also, it is so easy and quick to make.

## Energy Giving

It is an energizing food and will keep you active for a while after eating. It is healthier than other carbohydrate options, and delivers decent fibre too. It is a good meal option for diabetics, promotes the slow release of sugar into the bloodstream, and also keeps you full for a longer time.

### Did You Know?
Poha is gluten-free, so can be had by those allergic to gluten.

## Nutrient Load

Poha delivers some iron, which is much-needed in these times of rampant iron deficiency and falling haemoglobin levels. It also delivers B vitamins, particularly B1. The smartest thing about poha is that, traditionally, peanuts have always been added while making them, and they add some good quality protein and antioxidants, making the dish even more healthy. The lemon squeezed on top of the dish delivers vitamin C, which helps in better assimilation of the difficult-to-absorb iron (from vegetarian sources) from both the poha and peanuts.

## Go Experiment

Want an even healthier poha? Try poha made from red rice. The pigment anthocyanin (which gives it the colour) is an antioxidant and also delivers more fibre, vitamin B, calcium, zinc, iron, manganese and magnesium.

## Easy Tips to Eat Poha

For me, poha is a perfect food for enjoyment and energy. I love the traditional recipe (make it with lots of mustard seeds [rai], curry leaves, peanuts, potatoes and peas) and always eat it with a generous amount of lemon juice. I also like my red poha with lots of mushrooms, peppers and cheese (it tastes divine!) and I remember eating spinach poha often while growing up (an intelligent way of adding greens to a child's diet).

I think it is a smart move to add a protein source to poha (to make it a complete dish). Some options are tofu, sprouts and soya nuggets. They all combine well with poha. I know a lot of people who eat it with curd (instead of green chutney), and that is smart as well, as it makes the meal balanced and helps to get some calcium in the process.

One tempting concoction I had at a neighbour's house while growing up was made by soaking poha in water, sieving it, adding curd and a pinch of table salt in it, and then eating it with mango or lime pickle. I still remember that taste. In fact, during Makar Sankranti, a festival celebrating the arrival of spring and the change of season, dahi chura (curd poha) is very commonly eaten in many states in north India. In Mangaluru, they have poha paired with chickpeas (a grains-lentils combination), and Jains often stuff samosas with spicy poha.

Some have it sweet too. Doodh cheere, or rice flakes soaked in milk and mashed together with bananas, is a traditional breakfast favourite in West Bengal. A friend makes it like a pilaf by adding nuts, raisins and some sugar. Down south, they make a mean aval nanachathu (moist poha) with grated coconut, cardamom, milk and jaggery, and banana slices. In some southern temples, I have been told that aval (poha) also features as prasadam.

So, get poha back on the menu, and eat it more often, I say. If you need inspiration, go hotfoot to Krishna land and taste that yummy poha there.

## At a Glance

The benefits of eating poha include,

- Giving your stomach a break
- Stocking up on B vitamins
- Getting easily digestible energy
- Taking a gluten break
- Getting comforted

### Fun Fact
Poha may be rightly described as one of the world's first fast foods, which just happens to be super-healthy too!

Chapter 16

# FOX NUT

### The Fox Nut Foxtrot

Raise your hands if you feel like munching on something crunchy and salty and delicious with your cup of tea every evening! If you do, take my advice and instead of the disastrous chips or fried namkeen, snack on popped fox nuts (also called makhana). Not only will they satisfy you more, you'll do your body a lot of good too.

Not many people know that the underrated seeds of many plants are extremely delicious and healthy, and makhana are a perfect example of that. These seeds of Euryale ferox (and not the lotus plant, as commonly assumed), an aquatic flowering plant that grows in stagnant water in wetlands, have always been very popular during religious rituals in India and have been a prominent fasting food since ancient times. And all for good reason!

Lightly roasted in just a little bit of ghee and seasoned simply with salt and pepper (some add a bit of haldi too), this chameleon food that takes on the flavour of the seasoning added to it, is a great way to satisfy the cravings that undo most good diets.

It's loaded with fibre, so even eating a small amount of it satisfies our hunger pangs, and along with its perfect crunch, it delivers multiple nutrients that are super hard to find. I am a huge fan, and to me, every bite is sheer pleasure!

Need more convincing to include it in your diet? Read on.

## Low Glycemic Index

Makhana is a good source of protein and fibre, is moderately high in calories (50 gm will give you 175 calories) but as they are a low glycemic index food, they get digested slowly. And that makes them a better bet for diabetics over other crunchy snacks (yes, even popcorn).

## Tame Your Blood Pressure

Makhana helps keep our electrolyte balance and blood pressure in tandem as they are high in potassium but low in sodium (just don't add too much salt when you roast them).

## Gluten-free

Makhana is gluten-free, and so, great for people who are gluten intolerant and even for those who just want to eat gluten-free for a while to give their body a break. This is precisely the reason why makhana flour is much in demand these days.

## Reverse Ageing

Fox nuts deliver kaempferol (also found in tea, coffee, broccoli, bell pepper and cabbage), and antioxidants that helps cut inflammation and prevent ageing. For this reason, they are often called the age-locking, wrinkle-banishing seed. They also deliver phytonutrients, alkaloids, gallic acid and saponins, which protect us from common lifestyle disorders, and the high calcium in it helps keep our bones and teeth happy.

## Delivers Magnesium

It helps to know that magnesium is found to be lower in those suffering from unhappiness. Makhana delivers a lot of magnesium, so consuming them regularly can help keep us happier. This mineral also helps reduce heart attacks by relaxing the blood vessels. Makhana also delivers zinc, phosphorus and some calcium.

## The B1 Benefit

Makhana have vitamin B1 (thiamine), which is hard to find but plays a key role in nerve, muscle and heart function. They are the key to converting the carbohydrates we eat to energy in the body. Not getting enough B1 often leads to chronic fatigue. So, munching on a few fox nuts every day might help you stay charged all day. B1 deficiency has also been linked to vision trouble. Now we know why our grandmas used to tell us to eat these seeds for a super-sharp vision.

**Did You Know?**
Ayurveda and Unani medicine practitioners consider it an aphrodisiac and a boon for reproductive health.

## Banish Insomnia

Makhana has a sedative and calming function too, thanks to the isoquinoline alkaloids found in these seeds. They are also known to improve appetite and detoxify the body.

## Easy Tips to Eat Fox Nuts

There are multiple ways to eat makhana of course. You could dry roast them, or roast with a little ghee or coconut oil and flavour them with natural spices and condiments like mint leaves, curry leaves, coriander powder, garlic powder, turmeric powder, green chillies, etc.

They are perfect as a snack mix (just add some peanuts, cashews and/or almonds to them). Seasoned popped makhana is, of course, perfect. Try unusual flavours like wasabi, jalapeño, etc. to keep things interesting. I believe it is a perfect food to wean children (and even adults) away from processed, junk snacks.

I love to soak them overnight, and add them to salads, curries, pulao, raita and desserts. I grew up eating makhana kheer and even today, it is my comfort food.

## At a Glance

The benefits of eating makhana include,

- Tuning your body's electrolyte balance
- Preventing inflammation and ageing
- Ensuring good nerve health
- Giving a gluten holiday to your body
- Banishing wrinkles
- Keeping our heart and mind happy
- Fighting sleeplessness
- Staying supercharged and fatigue-free

### Fun Fact
Chinese have been using fox nuts as medicine for almost 3,000 years now.

Mini Chapter IV

## EASY HACKS

**Fixit Tip 43**: To make your soup even better, add at least one of these each time—garlic, onion or ginger—as these are natural antibiotics and immunity boosters.

**Fixit Tip 44:** Feeling rundown and low on energy? Maybe you need to boost your intake of CoQ10 (short for Coenzyme Q10). CoQ10 supplies cells with energy and also protects us from premature ageing. For this, eat 1 tbsp of sesame seeds (til) every day.

**Fixit Tip 45**: Tired? Take 3-4 dates and boil them with one glass of milk or water. Eat the dates and drink the milk or water. This gives instant energy, and hydrates effectively too.

**Fixit Tip 46:** Mix asafoetida (heeng) and dry ginger powder along with some honey and have this mix to get relief from respiratory issues.

**Fixit Tip 47:** Falling sick too often? Drink your lemons! It is the ideal food for restoring the acid-alkali balance and boosting healthy bacteria.

**Fixit Tip 48:** Gas trouble? Take ½ kg of uncrushed carom seeds (ajwain) and 20 gm each of rock salt, black salt and table salt. Mix all of these with a little lemon juice and keep for a few days till the mixture dries. Take ½ tsp of this with warm water every day.

**Fixit Tip 49:** Heartburn? Take a mixture of 1 tsp of cumin seeds and 1 tsp of carom seeds and add ½ tsp of ginger powder with water till the heartburn disappears.

**Fixit Tip 50:** Are you a vegetarian? Be 'C' smart. Pair spinach, pomegranate and chickpeas with vitamin C-rich foods (orange, lemon) to boost iron absorption.

**Fixit Tip 51:** Worried about not getting enough calcium? Figs are a brilliant source of calcium, a mineral that is essential for boosting bone density.

**Fixit Tip 52:** Is cough bothering you? Take equal quantities of black pepper seeds, long pepper seeds and dried ginger. Grind together to a fine powder. Make a paste of ¼ tsp of this mixture and a little honey, and have this paste 3–4 times a day to ease your cough.

**Fixit Tip 53:** To beat asthma-induced muscle spasms, add 1 tsp of carom seeds to a glassful of water and bring to a boil. Add ½ tsp washed, dried and home-ground turmeric powder to this. Simmer for 3–4 minutes on a low flame. Strain, add a pinch of salt, a little sugar or honey, and sip this as a herbal tea while still hot.

**Fixit Tip 54:** Feeling tired in the afternoons? Include one fermented food in your lunch to help good bacteria thrive in the intestines. This will help in better digestion of food and assimilation of nutrients, which ensures enough energy. Sprouts, dhokla, yoghurt, buttermilk and kanji are good options.

**Fixit Tip 55:** Want to stay alert? Fennel seeds-infused water works as a mild stimulant and sipping it throughout the day can keep you alert and awake. In fact, there is no need for any caffeine.

**Fixit Tip 56:** Does jet lag bother you? Fill your stomach with a high-carbohydrate snack (like a sandwich), and a drink containing electrolytes (like lemon water, coconut water, etc.) an hour before flying. This helps stabilize the blood pressure and prevent jet lag.

**Fixit Tip 57:** Donating blood? Begin eating iron-rich foods like prunes, figs and tomato juice, at least a week or two before the date. Having an iron-rich meal just on the day of donation does not help, as iron levels in the body take time to go up.

**Fixit Tip 58:** Having pomegranate today? Make sure you squeeze in some lemon, as vitamin C is essential for absorption of iron from pomegranate.

Similarly, always add some lemon juice or sweet lime (mosambi) juice to anar juice.

**Fixit Tip 59:** On a birth control pill? Go on a fig overdrive as the pill depletes vitamin B6 in the body and you need an extra dosage. B6 also helps produce mood-boosting serotonin in the body.

**Fixit Tip 60:** Have a citrus fruit juice (like orange or mausambi) rather than apple juice for breakfast—they have more vitamin C.

**Fixit Tip 61:** Feeling low? Eat some fennel seeds. It releases endorphins into the bloodstreams, which can lift up our mood and relieve depression too.

**Fixit Tip 62:** When eating out, ask for the bread basket to be removed from your table as soon as you sit down. Easiest way to cut down your carbs consumption!

**Fixit Tip 63:** Make a decoction of tea leaves, mint and a bit of ginger. Add a dash of honey and sip this hot to get relief from chest congestion.

**Fixit Tip 64:** Mix a tsp each of ginger juice and honey, warm it and drink just before sleeping to relieve severe cough (every night for a week).

**Fixit Tip 65:** A clove (laung) and a cardamom (dalchini) kept in the mouth while traveling helps keep motion sickness away.

**Fixit Tip 66:** To make dosas crispy, add soaked fenugreek seeds to the ingredients while grinding. You'll get some extra nutrients and antioxidants too.

**Fixit Tip 67:** Have a veggie juice instead of tea at 5 p.m. It'll help cut down your caffeine intake and also give you essential vitamins, minerals and antioxidants.

**Fixit Tip 68:** A good combination for an anytime snack: 1 tomato, some walnuts and a bit of feta cheese. It works wonderfully because you get some super powerful antioxidant lycopene, protein and some calcium too, all under 150 calories.

**Fixit Tip 69:** Midday blues? Sip a cup of warm holy basil (tulsi) tea and feel your stress melt away. Tulsi functions as an adaptogen, and decreases the stress hormone level in the body. Make a cuppa by infusing chopped tulsi leaves in boiling water for 8 minutes.

**Fixit Tip 70:** To help cut down salt from your diet, begin adding a little lemon zest. It will help balance out the flavour.

**Fixit Tip 71:** Add a handful of soaked beans or sprouts in your raita. It will give added nourishment, and make the raita tastier.

**Fixit Tip 72:** Tomatoes are a superfood, but do you want to know how to have more? Make tomato puree in bulk, freeze in ice cube trays, and store in a ziplock bag. Use whenever you want to.

**Fixit Tip 73:** Sprinkle wheatgerm over cereals, dahi and salads, or use it in muffins, cookies and pancakes; the fibre boost you get from wheatgerm is phenomenal.

**Fixit Tip 74:** Quit eating sugar-loaded, ready-to-eat jams and try this instead: Put some raw almonds, some water, a little honey, and a date into the mini-blender. In seconds, have a delicious spread for your toast.

Chapter 17

# GHEE

## Yes, that Dollop of Ghee Is Good

If you are one of those people who refuse to bow down to health fads and continue to include some ghee in your diet, then you should be glad because by doing so, you have done your body a lot of good. There's a lot that is good with this much-maligned fat source. Our ancestors always knew this, and gave ghee the importance it deserves—which is why it is customary in some Indian cultures to give a newborn a tiny taste of dates mixed with a little ghee! Unfortunately, ghee somehow got sidetracked along the way. But now, even the West is waking up to it, so it's time to remind everyone why we must include some ghee (a tsp or two) in our daily diet.

## Goodness Galore

Ghee delivers healthy fat-soluble vitamins like A, D, E and K, which our body needs regularly. Vitamin A is important to keep our eyesight sharp and our skin moisturized, vitamin D helps keep tiredness and aches away, vitamin E is imperative for heart health and without vitamin K, our bones will crumble.

It is now also clear that ghee, in spite of being a source of saturated fat, actually helps keep the serum cholesterol levels down and thus helps lower the risk of heart disease. In fact, there is no significant evidence about dietary saturated fat being associated with an increased risk of heart disease.

All this while, we have simply been blaming the wrong foods for our heart issues it seems—ghee included.

The oil that we use for cooking has a smoke point, i.e., the temperature at which fat begins to burn, an acrid smell abounds and a bluish smoke begins to emerge. Besides spoiling the taste of the food, this is the point when oils turn carcinogenic too. Cooking with ghee has no such worries as it has an extremely high smoke point; so, unlike most other fat sources, it does not form cancerous free radicals and also keeps inflammation in check even when heated to high temperatures. That's a huge boon!

One big problem most of us are facing today is the completely off-balance ratio of polyunsaturated fatty acids—Omega-6 and Omega-3—in our diet. Thanks to the overuse of vegetable oils, we are consuming way too much Omega-6, which increases inflammation (making us prone to myriad disorders) in the body. Ghee, fortunately, has an outstanding Omega-6:Omega-3 ratio, so it's far safer to consume that way.

Ayurveda has always maintained that ghee is good for the brain, making it sharper, and increasing memory retention. Modern science hasn't really caught up on this aspect yet, but hopefully, soon it will.

## Butyric Boost

Ghee (and actually even butter and cheese) delivers butyric acid, a short-chain fatty acid that acts as a detoxifier, improves colon health, aids digestion, boosts our immunity and also improves insulin sensitivity. In short, it is a wonder ingredient for our gastrointestinal system. There is enough evidence to show that most diseases originate in the gut—a diseased gut that is. There aren't too many foods that deliver butyric acid, so that is why ghee is priceless!

When sourced from grass-fed cows, ghee is a rich source of hard-to-find vitamin K2 (not found in leafy greens unlike K1). K2 helps put calcium where it should be (teeth and bones) and takes it out of places it shouldn't (arteries, kidneys, tissue, etc.). Remember the age-old saying that our elders didn't tire of repeating: Ghee feeds the bones! I wonder how they understood the connection! Perhaps by simple observation. Now scientists are studying to see if K2 has heart-friendly properties too.

### The Fit Fat!

You'll find it difficult to believe, but ghee can actually help you lose weight too, thanks to a high amount of the healthy fat, conjugated linoleic acid (CLA), an antioxidant with anti-viral and anti-weight gain properties. CLA particularly helps get rid of the weight around the abdomen, which is considered to be the most dangerous fat in the body as it can affect the heart. So you can discard the assumption that ghee makes you put on weight.

That is not all! Ghee can help cut cravings too. We all need to (but ignore) eat good fats as these are essential for building hormones in the body. They are especially important for keeping the level of the stress hormone, cortisol, low. High cortisol leads to conversion of blood sugar into fat for long-term storage (and thus weight gain). It also causes food cravings and addictions, frequent headaches, anxiety and irritability. Thus, including some ghee in your diet can actually help you stay thin.

### Did You Know?

Although ghee is derived from milk, it contains very low lactose, so it is perfectly okay even for people who are lactose intolerant. Also, it is the absence of milk solids and water in ghee that makes it shelf stable. That's why it stays okay even without refrigeration for long, unlike butter.

## Easy Tips to Eat Ghee

Finally, let's face it, ghee does add a lot of taste and flavour to food (a parantha tastes like a parantha only when made with some ghee, doesn't it?), and unless the food is tasty, it will never satisfy us. Of course, as with any other food, particularly with a highly calorific fat source like ghee, moderation is the key. So, go easy on it, but make sure you have some every day, like our forefathers did till some decades back.

## At a Glance

The benefits of eating ghee include,

- Deriving vitamins A, D, E and K
- Getting good fats
- Keeping cholesterol in check
- Cutting inflammation
- Boosting bone and brain health
- Providing butyric acid, which keeps the gut clean
- Deriving CLA, which helps keep weight and waist in control

### Fun Fact

Our ancestors in India discovered how to make ghee to preserve butter or cream, as they had no other means of preservation.

Chapter 18

# GREEN GRAM

## Why You Must Eat More of the Mighty Moong

Two honest questions: How often do you eat green gram (also known as moong dal, mung beans and peeli dal) in a week? And how much importance do you give it as a source of protein, energy, nutrients, etc.?

The fact is that most of us don't give it much thought. In fact, even as children we never tired of saying: 'Oh no, not moong dal again!'

Not surprisingly, they don't get written about much either, unlike say, chickpeas or kidney beans (rajma).

## On a Comeback Trail

But it seems certain people are giving this humble legume more than a passing thought and are touting it as a meat-free source of protein for everyone, not just vegans and environmentalists.

That's not all! The West has found a way to eat mung beans as protein powders and canned soups, and the legume is popping up in fancy restaurant dishes too. Unfortunately, we are not giving it the importance it deserves in India! Can't imagine moong dal replacing the popular kaali dal (dal makhani) anytime soon in restaurant menus!

But there are plenty of reasons to eat more of this ubiquitous dal–as it is plenty in supply here–and make it an intrinsic part of our meals again, just the way it was till a decade or two back.

## Easily Digestible

These legumes are cherished by Ayurveda experts, as this ancient science considers them tridoshic, which means that they work well for all body types when cooked with the right spices. My mom cooks moong very simply, mixing the whole and the split dal (after soaking for a few hours) with lots of ginger and a spice mix of cumin, coriander and turmeric, and it tastes delicious. These beans are one of the easiest to digest, and unlike most other beans, don't cause flatulence (formation of gas). They also help to detoxify the gut and the body.

The yellow moong dal (skinned green gram) is lighter and easier to digest. The famous Moradabadi Dal made of yellow moong has an interesting history. In 1625, one of the cooks of Prince Murad Baksh (the third son of Mughal king Shah Jahan) of Moradabad accidentally discovered that cooking moong dal on slow flame led to a dish that was slightly sweet, velvety and very flavourful. He served it in a bowl made of dried betel leaf, with a garnish of amchur, onions and green chillies. The prince apparently liked it so much that he snacked on it three times a day. And, thus, Moradabadi Dal was born.

### Did You Know?
Moong is a cooling food. Drinking the water in which green moong dal has been soaked overnight is actually a cooling superfood. That's because it contains antioxidants such as vitexin and isovitexin, which protect against the free radical damage that occurs during high temperatures and heat stroke.

## Nutrient Dense

Packed with lots of fibre, very good-quality protein, very low fat, lots of potassium, magnesium, folate, copper (which delivers powerful anti-ageing benefits) and vitamin B6, they are a power-food. When combined with whole grains, they deliver complete protein, and thus, are a boon for strict vegetarians and vegans.

## A Weight Watcher's Friend

Another good news is that because of the high level of protein and fibre, eating this dal leads to an increase in the satiety hormone called cholecystokinin, which helps one stay full for long and suppress hunger. So, if you are on a diet, snack on moong. They also deliver resistant starch–soluble, fermentable fibre–which boosts good bacteria in the gut.

## They Help Our Heart

Moong helps stop the oxidation of LDL 'bad' cholesterol, a huge risk factor for heart disease and stroke. Peptides present in mung beans and the high amount of magnesium in them, help ease blood vessels and lowers hypertension. So, those battling with blood pressure issues must give this dal a chance.

## Anti-inflammatory

The antioxidants found in moong help lower inflammation and thanks to their low glycemic index, they release sugar slowly in the body and display a significant anti-diabetic effect. Finally, high levels of amino acids, oligosaccharides and polyphenols make it a brilliant anti-cancer food too.

Now that's a bag full of reasons to begin cooking more of this simple dal.

## Easy Tips to Eat Green Gram

The dal can be cooked in a multitude of ways, and you can also get inventive and eat more of it, for your own good. Try this age-old recipe found classical Indian literature, when pulses were often blended with vegetables to prepare flavourful curries. Season moong dal with pieces of lotus stem, chironji seeds, asafoetida and green ginger, and then fry in oil and boil to a curry. Now add fried brinjal, and finish with black pepper and dry ginger.

Moong dal khichdi is India's favourite comfort food, and for good reason. Feed it to children by making a tangy mix and using it as a pizza base, or give them a spicy potato-moong-cucumber chaat. Mung beans can also be enjoyed sprouted, both raw and cooked. I often eat sprouted moong dal as a sandwich filling or make a cheela (soak and grind the sprouts; then season and add some veggies).

## At a Glance

The benefits of eating moong dal include,

- Lowering inflammation in the body
- Cutting bad cholesterol
- Staying full for longer
- Cooling the body from inside
- Boosting good bacteria

## Fun Fact

Folklore has it that a simple, nutritious and subtly flavoured mix of five lentils, or panchmel dal—moong, chana, toor, masoor and urad—was apparently one of the favourite dishes of Jodha Bai, the Rajput wife of Mughal king, Akbar.

Chapter 19

# GUAVA

## Why Guava is a Superfruit

Guava (amrood) has been around for ages and is loved by almost everyone. But its health benefits aren't understood that well, as also the fact that the amount of goodness packed in this easily available fruit makes it a bonafide superfruit. In fact, I think it is a really cool fruit.

It is super-low in calories—one fruit (about 50 gm) gives only about 40 calories and comes packed with lots of fibre (3 gm per fruit). That is why it lists high on the satiety index and can keep one full for long. What this means is that if you have a medium-sized guava right after your lunch, you will not feel hungry again until the evening. It could even keep you full till dinner. Water makes up to approximately 80 per cent of a guava, making it a super-hydrating food.

## Guava Goodness

The fibre in a guava helps keep our gut in good health, keeps constipation away, and also binds the cancer-causing chemicals and throws them out. The astringents in guava help keep stomach infections away. Guava helps slow down the absorption of sugar in the blood, and so, it is a diabetic-friendly fruit.

### The C Powerhouse

Guava is loaded with vitamin C and contains four times the amount present in oranges. Eat it with the peel though, as the flesh just underneath is packed with C.

So, what does vitamin C do for us? It is an effective immunity booster and helps maintain a high level of collagen, keeping our skin firmer and more elastic. It is a natural antihistamine, which is why vitamin C-rich foods are highly recommended to people with allergies or asthma.

### The A Advantage

The contents of vitamin A and lycopene are also huge in guava. In fact, a pink guava provides twice the amount of lycopene than what a superfood like tomato delivers. Lycopene prevents skin damage from UV rays and offer protection from prostate cancer too.

> **Did You Know?**
> Guava has ellagic acid, a natural antioxidant that has proven immunity-boosting and cancer-protecting qualities.

### Go Guava!

Guava also has a moderate source of B-complex vitamins such as B3 (niacin), B5 (pantothenic acid), B6 (pyridoxine), E and K, as well as difficult-to-find minerals like magnesium, copper and manganese. Magnesium in particular helps in relaxing our nerves and muscles and keeps us calm and happy, thus making guava a 'good mood' food. The copper in it helps regulate the production, absorption and regulation of the thyroid hormone. Guava also delivers lots of potassium, which is essential to control our heart rate and blood pressure.

## Easy Tips to Eat Guavas

This is a fruit to eat if you want complete health, and you want the taste along with the crunch. You can, of course, just bite into a fresh fruit, make a nice salad out of it, or cook with it. Make a guava soup or check out the guava curry recipe in the recipes section.

## At a Glance

The benefits of eating guava include,

- Getting good hydration
- Keeping thyroid glands healthy
- Staying relaxed and calm
- Protecting the skin from UV rays
- Preventing asthma and allergies

### Fun Fact
The skin of a guava can be green, yellow, cream, or red in colour, while the colour of the flesh may be white, yellow, red or pink.

Chapter 20

# INDIAN GOOSEBERRY

### The Incredible Indian Berry

Ignore this small berry at your own peril! After all, Ayurveda has vouched for the Indian gooseberry (amla) for a host of health benefits, from digestive health to easing cough, for ages now. The fruit, seed, leaves, root, bark and flowers are parts of the plant that are used in traditional Indian medicine. Today, modern science too supports all these claims and is endorsing amla's goodness wholeheartedly.

### Nutrition Punch

Amla is 80 per cent water, and has some proteins and carbohydrates, as well as loads of fibre. It also has minerals (calcium, copper, magnesium, phosphorous, potassium, zinc and iron) and vitamins (carotene; B vitamins like B1 [thiamine], B2 [riboflavin], B3 [niacin], B5 [pantothenic acid], B6 [pyridoxine] and B9 [folate]; vitamin C and vitamin E2). This berry is, in fact, packed with multiple antioxidants—it has 30 times more polyphenols than red wine and more ellagic and gallic acid (potent antioxidants) than any other fruit!

### C Powerhouse

Vitamin C is our best bet to boost our immunity and keep flu, cold and myriad other viruses at bay. And amla is the most concentrated plant source of vitamin C. This makes it a potent antioxidant food and a great immunity booster, besides helping improve absorption of iron and calcium from food. That is why it is a great idea to eat it or have it along with iron- and calcium-rich foods. Vitamin C and some astringents in amla also keep the gums healthy and ensure a fresher breath.

## Disease Healer

Amla's broad-spectrum antioxidants work effectively to slow the ageing process and help prevent the build-up of plaque in the arteries, thus keeping heart diseases at bay. It is a great hypolipidemic agent and can produce a significant reduction in total cholesterol, LDL, triglyceride and very-low-density lipoprotein (VLDL). It also has chromium, which helps reduce the LDL cholesterol content of the body, thus boosting our heart's health. In addition, it fortifies the lungs and helps detox our systems. Besides boosting our immunity, amla also helps increase the white blood cell count in the body, which is the main line of defence for the immune system.

## A Friend of Diabetics

Amla packs in difficult-to-find trace mineral chromium, which has therapeutic value for diabetics as it helps in boosting the secretion of insulin and thus, keeps fasting blood sugar levels in check.

## Liver Strengthener

Amla has mild diuretic properties, which means that it increases the frequency as well as amount of urination. This helps in eliminating excess water, salt and uric acid from the body. It also helps strengthen the liver and flushes out its toxins (accumulated deposits of preservatives and additives). So it is a perfect antidote to all that junk food you eat.

## Gut Health Enhancer

Amla is an alkaline food and helps balance the stomach acid level, making the gut alkaline. An alkaline gut is essential for overall health and vitality. Amla also alleviates the symptoms caused by indigestion, flatulence, etc.

**Did You Know?**
Amla is a boon for our eyesight. It has carotene, which strengthens our vision and prevents age-related degeneration.

## Beauty Aid

Amla is great for our skin and hair, thanks to its high iron and carotene content. The antioxidants it packs in help reign in free radicals that are known to cause damage to skin cells and hair follicles, leading to premature skin ageing and hair loss. It actually works against free radicals from the UVB radiation in sunlight, which breaks down the skin's connective collagen and leads to wrinkles and sagging skin.

## Oral Health Booster

As amla is such a powerful antimicrobial agent, it's great for our dental health too. Amla inhibits the growth of multiple bacteria and therefore, is beneficial as a treatment (and prevention) for dental caries, such as tooth decay and cavities.

## Easy Tips to Eat Indian Gooseberries

One amla a day is enough for our dietary requirements. You can grate the berry and add to subzis and salads, or just chomp on it.

Amla pickle is also very popular and so is amla murabba for those who prefer it sweet. You can drink it too—juice it or just boil it with a little salt and turmeric. Or you can just have some amla powder mixed with water or sprinkle it on a fruit—banana or papaya. To make the powder, dry the amla in shade for a few days and then grind it. Amla chutney and dried candies are fabulous too.

## At a Glance

The benefits of eating amla include,

- Scoring great skin
- Boosting immunity
- Making your gut alkaline
- Scoring antioxidants
- Detoxifying the liver
- Staving off heart disease

### Fun Fact
The amla fruit was considered so nourishing that its tree was worshipped in ancient India.

Mini Chapter IV

## FIX ESTROGEN IMBALANCE

**Fixit Tip 75:** The imbalance of the estrogen hormone shows up as abdominal obesity, bloating, cold hands and feet, hair loss, mental fogginess, hot flashes, night sweats and temperature swings. To fix it, have spirulina. It has essential fatty acids that help the liver to metabolize the excess estrogen. You can have it mixed with water or just add to smoothies.

**Fixit Tip 76:** To ease the symptoms of menopause, include foods that have a lot of phytoestrogens—plant compounds that are both mildly estrogenic and mimic the action of estrogen in the diet: leafy green vegetables, broccoli, cauliflower, cabbage, chickpeas, beans and lentils.

**Fixit Tip 77:** Grapes can be a woman's best friend because of the bioflavonoids they contain. Bioflavonoids help with estrogen replacement, and can help control symptoms of menopause, such as hot flashes, fatigue, irritability and mood swings.

Chapter 21

# JACKFRUIT

### Jack of all Fruits

Even though the jackfruit (kathal) looks a little weird (and unappetizing), it is important to develop a taste for this fibrous food because of the nutrition punch it delivers. And that shouldn't really be a problem, as its taste has been described as that of a pineapple crossed with a banana—and is quite nice actually! When cooked, it tastes like meat, but is way better for you.

### Nutrition Giant

This giant fruit is rich in vitamins A and C, calcium, potassium, iron, thiamin, riboflavin, niacin and magnesium, besides giving some protein and lots of fibre. A cup (150 gm) will give about 140 calories, 2.6 gm protein and 2.3 gm fibre.

### Cancer Fighter

Jackfruit has anti-cancer and anti-ageing properties, thanks to the lignans, isoflavones and saponins—all the phytonutrients it is loaded with. These help eliminate free radicals, which can cause cancer, from the body.

### Eye Tonic

It has abundant vitamin A and compounds like xanthin and lutein, which help maintain sharp eyes (and smooth skin) and also keep night blindness away.

## Tames Blood Pressure

Jackfruit is a good source of vitamin B6, as well as two minerals, potassium and magnesium; all these help regulate blood pressure.

## Diabetic-friendly

Jackfruit has a low glycemic index, which means that it helps keep glucose levels steady and is, thus, a diabetic-friendly food.

## Weight Loss Tool

Jackfruit is a natural weight loss-aiding food, if had the right way (not fried that is!). It is not high in calories, replenishes energy and revitalizes instantly. It also satisfies your hunger, thanks to its high fibre content and keeps you full for longer (besides keeping your digestion happy too). It also has a lot of the antioxidant resveratrol (made famous by wine), which helps trim inches off your trouble areas.

## Jack Up Your Nutrients

The magnesium content in jackfruit makes it a bone-friendly food (feed it to your children definitely), and also helps beat insomnia.

Being one of the few foods rich in the micro mineral, copper, ensures that it keeps the thyroid gland healthy.

Eating one serving of jackfruit supplies over one-third of our daily requirement of vitamin C, which helps boost our immunity and protects us from stroke, heart disease and cataract.

Jackfruit is also a rich source of iron and folic acid, which help in preventing anaemia and improving blood circulation in the body, and B vitamins such as thiamine and niacin, which help beat fatigue, stress, and muscle and nerve weakness.

**Did You Know?**
The seeds of ripe jackfruit are edible and very delicious when roasted or boiled in salted water. They are also made into flour.

## Easy Tips to Eat Jackfruits

Jackfruit is eaten world over. It is Bangladesh's national fruit. In Thailand, they even make a jackfruit pudding, and it is so well-loved in Sri Lanka that they smoke it and store it (for when it is not in season).

Usually, ripe jackfruit is eaten as a fruit (try it, it's absolutely delicious) and unripe jackfruit is prepared as a vegetable. It has a mild flavour, which melds well with a variety of seasonings and when cooked, soaks up the flavour like a sponge and takes on a meat-like texture, making it an excellent vegetarian substitute for meat. Mostly, it is eaten fried or as a curry (goes very well with the coconut flavour).

You can even try kathal ki biryani. This unusual biryani made with fried raw jackfruit pieces cooked with a delicious blend of spices and basmati rice is an addictive dish. To give it a contemporary twist, pair it with quinoa or couscous. You can also make kathal pickle.

It is actually an adaptable food, and can be dried or roasted and used in everything from soups to noodles, jams to juices, and even ice cream.

Most importantly, don't miss the jackfruit chips in Kerala. They are yummy! You can also try their popular dish, chakka vevichathu, or chakka puzhukku—jackfruit boiled, mashed and sautéed with mild spices like turmeric.

## At a Glance

The benefits of eating jackfruit include,

- Delivering anti-cancer and anti-ageing properties
- Strengthening your bones
- Keeping your thyroid gland healthy
- Taming your blood pressure
- Sleeping better
- Knocking off weight

### Fun Fact
The largest tree-borne fruit in the world, jackfruits can go up to 3 feet in length and 70 kg in weight.

Chapter 22

# MANGO

## Marvellous Mango

There has to be something right with mangoes for they have been a part of the diet in India for more than 4,000 years. Like most people I know, I too love my mango and eat them with abandon. I actually eat them straight off the peel, no dainty, pretty-looking cubes for me. That's how I have eaten mangoes as a child and continue to do so as an adult. And now I know that eating mangoes like this pays rich dividends as the concentration of the anti-cancer and anti-inflammatory antioxidants that mango is rich in is maximum just below the skin. So, eating it the old-fashioned way (my way!) is actually the best way to score maximum health benefits.

Mango is a perfect comfort food: Just tasting one makes you feel good. It does effectively chase away the blues. It has many advantages over other fruits. For starters, it has minimal fat and sodium, and zero cholesterol. It is not very steep in calories (about 120 calories for a medium-sized fruit), so it makes a perfect in-between snack or/and a delicious dessert.

## Gut-happy Food

Ever noticed how your constipation simply clears up during the mango season? That's because mango delivers lots of fibre (3 gm), and works like a natural laxative. It's in fact a brilliant gut food.

Also, it is an alkaline food that helps keep the pH of the body alkaline. An acidic body is a seat for disease, and eating mangoes can help check that effectively.

## Antioxidants Loaded

Mangoes are loaded with more beta-carotene than most other fruits—about 2164 IU in 200 gm. Beta-carotene gets converted into vitamin A in the body, which is needed for good eyesight, healthy lungs, bones and skin. Also, these powerful antioxidants are good for a healthy immune system and help repair cell damage.

Mango is also a great source of vitamin C, which again helps boost our immune system. It is rich in glutamine acid, a protein that improves our concentration and memory.

Ripe mangoes possess loads of phenolics (antioxidants), which have anti-cancer and anti-inflammatory properties.

You score loads of potassium too and our body needs potassium to help regulate blood pressure (thus keeping hypertension away).

**Did You Know?**
Even though mangoes are a rich source of fructose (a type of fruit sugar), they needn't be forbidden from a diabetic's diet. Just incorporate them safely and responsibly. It's safe as its glycemic load (a useful measure of the ability of a food to spike blood sugar and insulin levels) is low-medium. So, diabetics need not be scared of this fruit.

### Not Fattening

Finally, it is time to really bury the myth that mangoes can be fattening. Eating a mango has been shown to reduce the level of leptin hormone in the body, which affects our appetite. So, in effect, mangoes may help control blood sugar and cholesterol and also reduce body fat. Mango peel extracts are also known to inhibit fat cell formation, very similar to the action of resveratrol (the antioxidant found in red wine, grapes and peanuts).

All this from that tasty, juicy fruit? Not a bad deal at all!

So, whether or not you are on a weight-loss diet, I'd say one mango a day while it is in season is mandatory for everyone. There are enough reasons to enjoy this fruit, and the joy they give is just *one* of those!

### Easy Tips to Eat Mangoes

You can just bite in, of course. And I suggest you eat it the traditional way—with the peel—so that when you suck on the flesh, you can absorb some antioxidants from the skin as well.

Make mango lassi in a blender by combining 1 mango, 1 cup yoghurt, 1 tbsp honey, 2 dates and ice. Blend until smooth. Then pour into glasses and serve.

To make mango salsa, mix together mangoes, cucumber, finely chopped white onion, lime juice, orange juice, roughly chopped mint leaves, salt and pepper. It goes perfectly with nachos.

Also try this for breakfast some day: Put milk, chia seeds and honey in a jar and refrigerate it overnight. Add fresh mango puree or chopped mangoes to it the next morning and enjoy a healthy breakfast.

## At a Glance

The benefits of eating mangoes include,

- 🍃 Providing energy
- 🍃 Delivering potassium to keep your blood sugar under control
- 🍃 Providing fibre to keep your constipation away
- 🍃 Sharpening concentration and memory
- 🍃 Boosting immunity

### Fun Fact
Mangoes were first grown in India over 5,000 years ago. It is believed that Lord Buddha meditated under the cool shade of a mango tree.

Chapter 23

# MORINGA

## India's Most Potent Superfood

Sometimes, all we need to do is to look in our backyard to find the superfood we need to score health and combat modern-day diseases. And moringa is just that superfood. It has lately been giving foreign and exotic superfoods some serious competition.

The drumstick tree, also called miracle tree, has been a part of traditional Indian diet for ages now, thanks to the insane amount of nutrition it delivers. The leaves are where most of the nutrients are concentrated and moringa powder is made from these. The presence of around 90 nutrients in moringa has already been known, but there's a possibility that more will be identified. The word 'moringa' may have been derived from the Malayalam 'murinna', Tamil 'murungai' (meaning twisted pod), or Sinhalese 'muruṅga'.

## Go Ga-Ga over Moringa!

Moringa is full of vitamins and minerals: significant amounts of vitamins A, B, (folic acid, pyridoxine and riboflavin), C and E, calcium, manganese, magnesium, potassium, phosphorous, zinc and protein. It is a rare plant food that delivers all eight essential amino acids that our body needs, making it a perfect protein source for vegetarians looking to score complete protein.

### Anti-ageing

Traditionally, moringa has been used as a natural energy booster and fatigue reducer. It helps keep up our vitality, possibly because it is loaded with antioxidants—flavonoids, polyphenols and ascorbic acid—which help purge free radicals from the body, which cause ageing. It also delivers quercetin, which cuts inflammation in the body, and chlorogenic acid, which has been shown to slow the absorption of sugar in cells, thus helping lower blood sugar. This makes moringa an effective anti-diabetic food.

### Cuts Inflammation

Moringa suppresses the action of inflammatory enzymes and proteins in the body, and helps keep chronic diseases like diabetes, respiratory problems, cardiovascular disease, arthritis, and obesity (which occur due to inflammation) at bay. It is a known liver cleanser too.

### Unique Advantages

This unique food helps to reduce both sugar and lipid levels in the body. It is great for our heart, as besides helping with blood lipid control, it also helps prevent plaque formation in the arteries, and cuts cholesterol.

Chlorogenic acid, which is present in a huge quantity in moringa, helps lower blood sugar by slowing the absorption of sugar in our cells, making it an effective anti-diabetic food. It also contains compounds like niaziminin, which are known cancer cell inhibitors.

### Brain Booster

A high content of vitamins E and C in moringa is great news for our brain as these help prevent cognitive decline. It helps to prevent Alzheimer's and also to ups the neurotransmitters serotonin, dopamine and noradrenaline, which boosts our memory and mood.

**Did You Know?**
Moringa is a natural beauty tool as the nutrients in it deliver healthy, glowing skin and stronger hair. Moringa leaves also purify the blood and naturally help in acne reduction.

## Stress-fighting Superherb

Moringa rightfully belongs to the niche group of adaptogens, the new stress-fighting superherbs, which have the nutrition world excited all over. Adaptogens are plants that effectively help the body adapt to stress and prevent it from running us down. They also help strengthen, rebuild and nourish our body. Moringa tops the list of adaptogens!

## Easy Tips to Eat Moringa

Fresh moringa leaves can be cooked in the same way as spinach and other leafy vegetables. If you have access to them, cook them fresh or have the powder or flakes. The best news here is that you need very little—about 3 gm of powder or about ¼ cup of fresh leaves per day—to score the benefits. Just blend fresh leaves with water and add some lemon juice and honey.

It tastes earthy and grassy, so to mask the taste, you can add some honey, maple syrup or cinnamon too, but make sure to have it either way for the unlimited benefits it delivers.

Some ways to eat moringa are:

i. Add the powder to watermelon chunks and some water, blend it and drink. You can also add it to your smoothie, cereal, soups and stews.
ii. Take half a mango, 1 banana, 1 tsp moringa powder and a few chunks of ice cubes; blend and sip.
iii. Put ½ tsp turmeric in a pressure cooker, and add a handful of moringa leaves and 2 glasses of water. Grind ½ tsp cumin seeds and 10 peppercorns and add to the cooker. Add 2 crushed garlic cloves and salt to taste. Cook the mixture till about three whistles. Strain the juice from the mixture, blend the residue in a mixer, strain again and mix with the juice strained earlier.

**At a Glance**

The benefits of eating moringa include,

- Scoring high-quality protein
- Delaying ageing
- Cutting inflammation in the body
- Preventing Alzheimer's
- Keeping blood sugar in check
- Boosting memory and mood
- For glowing skin and strong hair

**Fun Fact**
Moringa is a complete meal in a tree. All its parts—leaves, seeds and roots—are edible.

Chapter 24

# MUSHROOM

### I Love Mushrooms, and You Should too

Egyptian pharaohs prized mushrooms as a delicacy and the ancient Greeks and Romans fed them to their warriors. But why would someone even want to eat fungi?

It seems that all three civilizations had it right, as these potent fungi are both tasty as well as super-healthy. In fact, they are one of the healthiest ingredients you can plate to give your body a health boost.

### The Fantastic Fungus

Extremely nutrient-dense, mushrooms are low in calories (100 gm gives only 34 calories), are fat- and cholesterol-free, and are low in sodium and high in potassium; in fact, they outrank even bananas on the potassium chart.

Also, they provide complete protein (one of those rare vegetarian sources that delivers all essential amino acids) and decent fibre (2.5 gm per 100 gm), and there is an overload of vitamins and minerals too, most notable of which are vitamins C and B-complex, zinc, copper, manganese and the difficult-to-find antioxidant selenium. They are, in fact, a rare vegetable source of the critical vitamin D. So, there's a lot packed inside their rubbery texture.

## Antioxidants Overload

When it comes to antioxidants, mushrooms beat even colourful veggies like green peppers, carrots, green beans and tomatoes! They are loaded with a powerful anti-inflammatory micronutrient called ergothioneine, which gets released from the mushroom cells and becomes available when cooked. In fact, most of its nutrients remain stable even when cooked (unlike many other veggies). Mushrooms are, in fact, the richest source of ergothioneine, which acts as a cell protector. The human body cannot make erogothioneine, so you can get it from mushrooms (and also black beans).

## Immunity Booster

Freely eat mushrooms as these fungi promote the growth of white blood cells and make your body fighting fit. Mushrooms are easily digestible, help ease stomach ailments and eliminate food stagnation. They are also a probiotic food and help strengthen the body by upping its natural resistance to diseases. They are high in zinc too, which adds power to the disease fighters—white blood cells. When our immunity is robust, cancer and infections cannot sneak in.

## A Weight Loss Tool

Our metabolism relies on a healthy dose of protein, fibre and vitamin B to keep it functional and robust. Mushrooms deliver loads of these metabolism-supporting nutrients. They also deliver vitamins B2 (riboflavin) and B3 (niacin), which help boost our body's metabolism and help us lose weight faster. Their high fibre content and low calories also help fill us up with minimum calorie damage and loads of satiety.

**Did You Know?**
Mushrooms are said to help uplift us spiritually by calming and supporting nerve function.
They are also helpful for people who suffer from chronic stress, anxiety or insomnia.
So eat mushrooms and be happy!

### There's More!

They are a liver tonic too. They have a healing impact on the lungs and help keep asthma and respiratory issues in check. They also contain compounds that aid in the effective working of the pancreas, and this makes them a great food for diabetics. Now, in fact, they are being studied for their effect against AIDS too.

### Easy Tips to Eat Mushrooms

Most of us find it difficult to develop a taste for mushrooms! Agreed that the food seems a little alien, and the texture and taste are both a little different from the other vegetables we are used to eating day in and day out. However, trust me, it's time to change that, because ignoring this humble food means giving the multiple health benefits it packs within it a miss.

I like to have them simply stir-fried to chewy consistency at least twice a week. I also love to eat this mushroom toast: Just heat 2 tsp olive oil, add 2 garlic cloves and sauté for half a minute, then add chopped mushrooms and cook till they are done (about 5 minutes); season according to taste, place on a multigrain toast and dig in.

You can find your own way of incorporating them in your meals. Simply sauté and add to soups, sauces, salads and pizzas. Try to have different kinds of edible mushrooms as the benefits vary.

**TIP**
Next time you are thinking of making a meat dish, replace the meat with mushrooms. The texture is similar and you'll manage to cut loads of calories, salt and saturated fat with this one masterstroke.

## At a Glance

The benefits of eating mushrooms include,

- Slaying cancer
- Controlling cholesterol
- Uplifting your mood
- Strengthening the respiratory tract and liver
- Boosting the metabolism
- Upping the immunity

**Fun Fact**
Truffles, the mushrooms that grow below the ground, are one of the world's most expensive foods.

## Mini Chapter V

### SLEEP BETTER

**Fixit Tip 78:** Wind up your day with peppermint tea, some divine cheese and a couple of walnuts—all three are effective sleeping aids. This is actually a perfect sleep- and calm-inducing kit. Peppermint tea is relaxing and cheese works the same way as milk—it has calcium, which helps the brain to calm down using the tryptophan found in dairy, while walnuts help regulate the sleep cycle, thus helping one sleep better.

**Fixit Tip 79:** Is insomnia bothering you? Cumin seeds help relieve sleeplessness. Take 1 tsp roasted cumin seeds mixed with the pulp of a ripe banana at night to induce sleep.

Chapter 25

# ORANGE

### The Juicy Orange Wonder

This juicy, round, segmented, citrus fruit with a pitted peel has a taste that can vary from sweet to bitter, depending on the variety. However, one fact that stays common is that it is as nutritionally stacked as it is tasty. Oranges are loaded with vitamins A, B (including vitamin B1 and folate) and C, calcium and potassium. And one orange only gives 50–60 calories with a whopping 3.4 gm fibre.

### Bring on the C

One orange comfortably meets your daily vitamin C requirement, which helps sharpen your immune system, prevents oxidation of cholesterol (thus keeping your heart healthy), and reins in free radicals to prevent inflammatory disorders like asthma and arthritis. However, make sure you eat up the orange quickly once peeled, as exposure to air destroys the vitamin C.

### Anti-ageing

Orange is a very powerful anti-ageing food. The secret lies in its high vitamin C content, which is an effective antioxidant. Vitamin C also helps the body produce glutathione, a liver compound that drives away toxins and detoxes this important organ.

## Skin Care

This juicy tasty fruit is a boon for our skin, especially for those who have trouble with acne. The citric acid they have helps dry the acne. The vitamin C that orange has also helps prevent premature ageing of the skin due to free radicals by neutralizing them. It is also important for the production of collagen (the protein fibres of the skin). Collagen breakdown, which starts speeding up significantly around the age of 35, can leave your skin looking haggard. Flimsy collagen shows up as lines and wrinkles. Oranges, therefore, help prevent premature skin sagging.

Vitamin C also prevents the formation of pigmentation and bruises on the skin and helps keep up its elasticity.

## Lowers the Blood Pressure

Hesperidin, a flavonoid in orange, helps to keep blood pressure low (and cholesterol in check) and magnesium pitches in too. But instead of juicing it, go for the whole fruit as most of this flavonoid is found in its peel and inner white pulp. Also, to maximize the benefits of antioxidants, choose fully ripened oranges.

## Fibre+

The natural fruit sugar, fructose, in oranges helps keep the blood sugar from spiking; also it is loaded with fibre, so is great for diabetics too. The fibre also helps eliminate cancer-causing chemicals; thus, reducing the risk of colon cancer.

**Did You Know?**
After chocolate and vanilla, orange is the world's most favourite flavour.

## The Peel Advantage

While oranges are a minefield of antioxidants, its peel is specially loaded with hesperidin, which helps lower blood pressure and tame LDL cholesterol. Also, the compounds called polymethoxylated flavones (PMFs) found in these peels have the potential to lower cholesterol very effectively.

## Easy Tips to Eat Oranges

Orange is a portable fruit so you can have it while running errands around town or in between meetings. Juice it or add the segments to salads. Make salad dressings with it or add it to your bakes.

Also, don't just throw the peel away, add the zest to your smoothies, salads, soups and stir-fries, or brew a tea with it. You can even add some zest to other juices.

## At a Glance

The benefits of eating oranges include,

- Scoring younger-looking skin
- Boosting immunity
- Preventing acne
- Strengthening the liver
- Detoxifying the body

**Fun Fact**
Till the end of the nineteenth century, oranges were very expensive and were eaten only during special occasions like Christmas.

Chapter 26

# PAPAYA

### Papaya Power

How many of us have grown up seeing our parents eat a serving of papaya every day? Most of us, right? That fruit was a constant, while the others eaten during the course of a day would keep changing with the season. Papaya has been held in very high esteem, all thanks to the multiple benefits that it delivers.

I heard my grandmother often say that one doesn't need anything else to keep one's digestion in good shape. And yes, she used to eat it every single day. In fact, this universal and extremely versatile fruit, native to southern Mexico, is loved all over the world for its sweet taste with a musky undertone. It is also one of the most nutritionally loaded and healthy foods around—a fact that its sweetness often does not give away.

### Nutrition Punch

150 gm of papaya will give you only 60 calories and that's a steal for the nutrients it provides—fibre, potassium, and vitamins A, C, E, K and the B-family, including folate (vitamin B9). It also provides minerals like magnesium, calcium, phosphorous, iron and manganese, as well as a number of phytochemicals, carotenoids and other antioxidant compounds that help prevent ageing and the onset of lifestyle diseases. It is one of the most nutritionally loaded foods around, per-calorie.

## Immunity Boost

Vitamins A, C and E in papaya will keep your immune system really pumped up. It is a big help if one wants to keep recurring ear infections, colds and flus away. While many people know that papayas deliver lots of vitamin C, not many know that they also contain substantial amounts of folic acid and a generous portion of iron, both of which help combat anaemia and keep fatigue, shortness of breath, dizziness and headaches away. So, you just feel and function better with a daily dose of papaya.

## Digestive Agent

My grandma knew it instinctively, but now we also know that it is the enzymes–papain and chymopapain–in papaya that help break the protein that we eat, into amino acids. This helps prevent gastro distress and constipation. It also does a bigger job, as undigested protein not just leads to overgrowth of bad bacteria in our intestines, but also a shortfall of essential amino acids that our body needs a regular supply of. In fact, if the protein in our diet is not digested properly, it may in the long run even lead to arthritis, chronic constipation, piles, high blood pressure and multiple other health issues.

There's more. The presence of folate and vitamins C and E in papayas also reduces motion sickness naturally. So those who face this issue, now you know what to eat before you embark on long journeys.

## Anti-inflammatory

Papain and chymopapain also help reduce inflammation in different parts of the body. That makes papaya great for our bones too, as its anti-inflammatory properties, along with the vitamin C it has, helps in keeping various forms of arthritis at bay. The reduction of inflammation reduces pain at the joints. In fact, chymopapain has been found to have a significant effect on controlling both rheumatoid arthritis and osteoarthritis. Papaya also contains potassium, which helps keep the bones strong, and the presence of vitamin K helps the bones to get calcium directly. Those with a family history of arthritis and other bone-related issues must include this superfruit in their diet without a second thought.

## Lung Strengthener

In today's polluted times, this fruit can be a saviour. That's because papaya promotes lung health, thanks to the presence of vitamin A. Smokers and even those exposed to second-hand smoke tend to be extremely deficient in vitamin A, and prone to lung inflammation too, so they will specifically benefit by eating platefuls of this delicious fruit.

## Your Beauty Aid

Vitamins C and E, and carotenoids like beta-carotene and lycopene in papaya protect the skin from free radical damage, keeping wrinkles and other signs of ageing at bay. They also act as a natural 'sunscreen,' protecting the skin from harmful rays and therefore, preventing premature wrinkling. So, eating papaya is the secret to great skin.

Thanks to being an incredible source of minerals and vitamins, papaya also promotes hair growth and prevents hair fall. Vitamin A helps to enhance the production of sebum and as a result, also promotes hair growth, moisturizes your hair, and keeps it looking great.

## Eye Tonic

Carotenoids, lutein and zeaxanthin found in papaya protect the retina of the eye. The orange colour of papaya is due to its beta-carotene content, which gets converted into vitamin A in the body, and helps prevent macular degeneration (age-related vision problems).

## Hearty Powerfruit

The folate present in papaya helps control homocysteine in the bloodstream (a high level of homocysteine damages blood vessels and leads to heart disease), and the fibre in it inhibits the absorption of LDL cholesterol levels in the blood to keep its level low. Also, potassium—the legendary vasodilator—helps relieve the strain on the cardiovascular system by easing the tension in blood vessels and promoting better circulation, helping to keep blood pressure in check.

## Strengthen the Nerves

A high level of copper is important to help our nervous system to effectively communicate with other parts of the body. And a significant level of copper is found in papaya.

### Did You Know?
The enzyme papain found in papaya boosts the digestive process and increases nutrient absorption from protein-based foods.

## The Seeds and Leaves

Not many know that the small black seeds located at the centre of the papaya, with a very distinct spicy, peppery taste, are edible too. You can grind or just boil them to treat respiratory problems and purge intestinal worms. Papaya leaves are also helpful in treating the symptoms of dengue fever.

### Easy Tips to Eat Papayas

You can, of course, have a raw, ripe papaya, make a smoothie with it or cook, and make a subzi out of the slightly unripe ones. They are so versatile that you can incorporate them in your breakfast, lunch, snacks, or even have them for dessert! For a quick breakfast, just blend Greek yoghurt (or regular yoghurt), vanilla extract or cocoa powder, a frozen banana and a sliced, ripe papaya. For lunch, make this salad: Mix raw papayas, diced pineapple, garlic, lime juice, salt and black pepper.

### At a Glance

The benefits of eating papaya include,

- Saving your eyes from age-related degeneration
- Keeping your gastrointestinal system happy
- Keeping wrinkles and other signs of ageing at bay, and your hair lustrous
- Boosting your immunity
- Keeping your bones and joints super-strong
- Promoting lung health

#### Fun Fact
Papaya has many different fun names, like 'pawpaw' in Europe and Australia, 'fruta bomba' in Cuba, and 'mamão' in Brazil.

Chapter 27

# PEANUT

## Peanuts for Your Health

I get a lot of almonds and walnuts as Diwali gifts. Some enterprising people even gift roasted macadamia nuts and I am grateful to everyone as I sincerely believe that nuts make for a very healthy gift, be it for Diwali, Christmas, a wedding or even a birthday.

But this also got me thinking whether nuts are also graded—almost like the caste system! There are 'elite' nuts and then there are nuts that are considered 'poor cousins', regardless of how good they might be. And peanuts unfortunately have been relegated to the second category. Have you seen anyone gift peanuts, ever? Now this bothers me, as I believe these humble nuts belong right at the top in terms of what they deliver. There's no denying their delicious crunchy taste and texture, and they totally ace the nutrients front too. In fact, they deliver more than most other foods (even nuts) I know of.

## Protein Powerhouse

There is no doubt that peanuts are a cheap source of good quality protein. 30 gm of peanuts give you about 160 calories and 7 gm of protein, comparable to almonds, which deliver the same amount of calories and 6 gm of protein. Also, peanuts actually offer the best bang for the buck. Compare the costs with any other nut and you'll agree with me. They also deliver much more arginine than any other nut, an amino acid that delivers immunity and heart health. Arginine leads to the formation of nitric oxide, which prevents clotting by widening and relaxing blood vessels and thus, helping prevent heart attacks.

## A Bonafide Heart Food

Agreed that peanuts are high in fat but they are still very good for our heart. That is because the kind of fat that peanuts have is mostly monounsaturated fatty acids, which help reduce bad cholesterol. In addition, peanuts also deliver the heart-friendly antioxidant vitamin E; folic acid, which aids in reducing homocysteine, a risk factor; and plant fibre, which effectively cuts cholesterol.

## Better than Wine

Do you know the compound that made wine so popular the world over? Well, it is resveratrol. But here's an eye-opener: An ounce of red wine contains about 160 micrograms of resveratrol and 2 ounces of peanuts deliver the same amount. Resveratrol is definitely a wonder compound: It keeps our heart healthy, helps reduce the risk of cancer and delays ageing. Peanuts are even more wondrous because they also deliver folic acid, phytosterols and phytic acid, all anti-ageing compounds, as well as loads of niacin, which, combined with resveratrol, helps prevent the dreaded Alzheimer's disease.

### Did You Know?
Like olive oil, peanuts also deliver oleic acid. This good fat helps cut bad cholesterol in the body, fight inflammation and is excellent for the skin.

## Antioxidants Galore

Peanuts score very high on the antioxidants index. They are as rich in antioxidants as many fruits, and not many know that they deliver a similar amount as the much-hyped blackberries and strawberries, and much more than the very popular apples, carrots and beets.

## Easy Tips to Eat Peanuts

So, my suggestion is that don't ignore peanuts; eat them and gift them too. Put them everywhere—in the cakes and cookies you bake, in your soups and salads—or make a sauce or butter with them. And of course, add them liberally to your poha, upma or curd rice. Make munching on a few roasted nuts every afternoon a habit too. Move them higher in your grade if you haven't already, and give them the respect they deserve.

## At a Glance

The benefits of eating peanuts include,

- Scoring high-quality protein
- Boosting immunity and heart health
- Preventing Alzheimer's
- Cutting cholesterol
- Delaying ageing

### Fun Fact
Peanuts are actually not nuts. They belong to the legumes family.

Chapter 28

# PEAR

### Pears Are for All

Called 'nashpati' in our part of the world, pears are absolutely delicious. Their melt-in-the-mouth texture is easy to love. They are also the most unsung fruits around, but I'll give you five solid reasons to eat more of this delicious food.

### Heart Care

Pears are great for our heart (no cholesterol, no sodium and no saturated fats). They help bring down the bad cholesterol, thanks to the flavonoids they are packed with. In fact, eating two pears a day will ensure that your heart health is sorted, as they'll help you score the total flavonoids you need every day. They are a good source of potassium (119 mg) too, which keeps our blood pressure tamed—more good news for our hearts.

### The C Link

Pears deliver a lot of vitamin C, which helps cut the ill effects of pollution and eating too much junk. That obviously does not mean that you have a burger and then a pear and all will be good! But they can definitely help negate the damage and keep our immunity intact. The Chinese, in fact, consider pear, which they call 'li', a symbol of immortality. This may be because pear trees live for a long time.

## Quick, Healthy Energy

Pears are deliciously sweet and rightly so, as levulose, the sweetest of all known sugars, is found much more in this juicy fruit compared to other fruits. They also deliver large amounts of natural fructose and glucose, making them a quick source of healthy, tasty energy.

**Did You Know?**
Pears are a perfect means for diabetics to satisfy their sweet tooth as their abundant fibre helps keep blood sugar stable.

## Pearfect Snack

The best news is that in spite of being sweet, they are low in calories. A medium-sized (100 gm) pear provides just 60 calories and 3 gm of fibre. A large pear delivers just 100 calories with a whopping 5 gm of fibre. So it is a great weight loss tool and is perfect for snacking. Also, it is safe for everyone as pears are considered to be a hypoallergenic fruit; pear allergies being extremely rare. You will also hardly ever get an upset stomach when you eat a pear because its low acid level makes it very gentle on the digestive system. That's probably why ancient Greeks used it as a remedy against nausea.

## The Fibre Facts

The skin of a pear is soft and sweet, so it is usually eaten whole (without peeling) and that helps boost the fibre intake of this already high-fibre fruit. Fibre keeps our digestion working well, and cuts bad cholesterol and the risk of heart disease. Also, like apples, the antioxidant quercertin, which helps prevent cancer, heart disease and ageing, is found in the skin of pears.

## Easy Tips to Eat Pears

In China, it is considered bad luck for lovers or friends to share a pear because it may result in a quarrel or separation; interestingly, 'li' also means separation. But that aside, eating pear more regularly should be on everyone's agenda. Just bite in, or chop and toss into salads to add a sweet flavour, or have them stewed in various condiments for a fancy dessert. You could even poach one in wine—and get a double dose of antioxidants.

## At a Glance

The benefits of eating pears include,

- Cutting cholesterol levels
- Snacking right
- Getting quick, healthy energy
- Protecting yourself from pollution
- Lowering blood pressure

### Fun Fact
The Greeks were all about their pears! It was sacred to Hera and Aphrodite, goddesses in Greek mythology.

Mini Chapter VI

## HANGOVER CURES

**Fixit Tip 80:** Are you hungover? Have honey! Fructose (a readily absorbed form of fruit sugar) helps increase the rate at which alcohol is processed in the body. Eat 1 tbsp, or add some to water or a cup of tea. You can even spread some on wholewheat toast—the complex carbohydrates (found in the toast) will help neutralize an acidic stomach, while the simple carbs of honey will boost your energy fast, and help deal with lethargy.

**Fixit Tip 81:** Drank too much the previous day and plan to drink again today?

Have 2 slightly crushed cloves of raw garlic every day to score an amino acid called S-Allyl Cysteine, which'll neutralize acetaldehyde, a terrible byproduct of alcohol metabolism, and keep damages in check.

**Fixit Tip 82:** Eat peanuts while drinking alcohol; the niacin (vitamin B3) in peanuts helps break down alcohol in the body. They deliver tryptophan too, which converts into B3 in the body. Regular alcohol drinkers are often deficient in B3, which could lead to brain degeneration and dementia.

FIX IT WITH FOOD

Chapter 29

# PINEAPPLE

### Pile on the Pineapple

During a change in season, if you become a magnet for cold and flu attacks (don't we all, these days?) then an easy and tasty way to give your immunity a boost is by eating pineapples regularly. That's because of the two warriors that it has in its arsenal—the enzyme bromelain and loads of vitamin C—which help reduce inflammation of the nasal cavity and get rid of excessive mucus from the respiratory system, thus helping combat (and even keeping away) regular colds, coughs, and even bronchitis.

Unfortunately though, the only time most of us eat pineapples is when we order the Hawaiian pizza, or maybe drink a piña colada. I do know a few people who eat it regularly (a friend has a slice or two every day, in fact), but their number is very low. This fruit is really underrated despite the kind of benefits it bestows, and mostly gets overshadowed by other more commonly written about (hence, eaten) fruits likes bananas, berries and pears.

It's time to change that!

### Keep Disease Away

Pineapples are loaded with antioxidants, which have restorative and free radical-fighting properties, so it is particularly great to have when you are sick. Bromelain helps reduce inflammation, swelling, bruising and pain in the body. That's why it is often advised after surgery or injury to help reduce the trauma associated with incisions, injections and wounds. Similarly, it can help with a faster recovery from damaged muscle tissue and inflammations caused by strenuous exercise. So, those who exercise extensively must have their daily dose of pineapple. It is in fact a preventive tool too, as antioxidants help cut free radicals in the body, which cause chronic inflammation and a weakened immune system.

**Did You Know?**
Children who eat pineapples have a significantly lower risk of both viral and bacterial infections. This applies to adults too!

## Reduce bloating

It is a de-bloating food, as it is loaded with minerals (potassium) and enzymes that help cut the bloat and detoxify the body. There are three easy ways to have it.

Try this simple smoothie: Cut ½ cup pineapple, ½ cup papaya, 1 frozen banana, ¼ cucumber (with skin) into small pieces, add 1 cup chilled coconut water, blend and voila, you have your smoothie ready!

You can even have a green smoothie (spinach with pineapple and ginger); or juice 2 cups of fresh pineapple chunks, 1 small beetroot and ½ a lemon, and top it off by adding a pinch of salt.

## Clean-up Agent

Bromelain, an enzyme with anti-inflammatory properties, is mostly found in pineapple. It is a proven anti-cancer agent, which helps clean up our damaged cells and pollution-filled lungs.

## The C Advantage

Pineapples contain vitamin C which, besides being an immunity booster, also helps protect our vision and prevents cataracts. Enough vitamin C in our diet improves the quality of our skin and makes it radiant.

## There's More!

This juicy fruit delivers beta-carotene, copper, zinc and folate, which help boost fertility both in men and women. It also has high amounts of trace mineral manganese, which is needed for a healthy metabolism and strong bones, and thiamin, a B vitamin that is imperative for energy production in the body.

## No, It Won't Make You Fat

Finally, here's one myth that I really want to bust. Many people don't eat this sweet fruit thinking 'sweet' equals 'high in calories', but the fact is that 250 gm of pineapple gives only 125 calories and even though its glycemic index is 66, which some consider high, it is so loaded in fibre that its glycemic load (which is what matters actually!) is only 6. So, please feel free to have it; it won't make you fat. In fact, my experience as a weight management practitioner has taught me that a slice or two goes a long way in helping curb your cravings for sweets. A tasty way to stay thin!

## Easy Tips to Eat Pineapples

Avoid pineapples when the skin is still green, as it might cause acidity. Also, the unripe ones can be toxic, and may cause an upset stomach and throat irritation. When it is ripe and golden in colour though, this precious fruit is alkaline, which is great for realigning our gut's pH balance.

The Hawaiian pizza, a popular pizza variety with pineapple as a topping, was invented by a Canadian restaurant in 1962 and that's the only way most people I know eat the pineapple. Don't restrict yourself to a smattering however; find ways to have more of it. It is great as part of a fruit salad, or you can pair its slices with walnuts and snack on them. You can cook and eat it too. Try pineapple pulao, and chilled melon and pineapple soup.

Also, have you tried blending crushed pineapple pieces with cottage cheese for a sweet spread on your toast? It is quite divine!

## At a Glance

The benefits of eating pineapple include,

- Keeping cataracts away
- Preventing seasonal flus and viruses
- Speedily recovering from surgery or excessive exercise
- Curbing sweet cravings
- Boosting fertility

**Fun Fact**
Pineapples originated in South America, where early European explorers named it so, because of its resemblance to a pinecone.

Chapter 30

# POTATO

## Stop Maligning Potatoes, Start Eating Them

Potatoes (aloo) have been around since forever. They are versatile, and even though this may surprise you, they are healthy too. That is why I don't understand from where the hate for potato stems from. I love them, eat them often and you should too.

### A Versatile Food

First, they are extremely versatile. They can be served any time of the day—breakfast, lunch, dinner and snacks. They can be baked, roasted, boiled, steamed or fried, and can be fixed any which way you want—stand alone, added with any veggies, curried or dry; there are thousands of popular aloo recipes floating about. In fact, they pair well with just about any other ingredient. Don't fancy broccoli? Make a cheesy broccoli and potato soup. Similarly, spicy potatoes with bitter gourd can make the latter more palatable.

### Cook Them Right

In this case, the food itself is not the devil. How you cook them—a healthy low-calorie recipe or sinfully fried—is what matters. They usually get messed up (and become bad for us) because of how we cook them. When we add butter to mashed potatoes, we add up to 100 calories per tbsp, and every ounce of cheese increases the calorie count of the dish by 120 calories. Simple changes like opting for sour cream (at 20 calories per tbsp) or cream cheese (at 50 calories) are better bets. So, when you load potatoes with butter, cheese or bacon, or deep fry them, please don't blame the potato.

## A Great Choice

Potatoes may be the quintessential carb—a taboo in some dieting circles; in fact, it is the first food that goes out of the window when the urge to diet strikes—but the truth is that it is actually a great choice. One medium potato (150 gm) gives you about 116 calories and 3 gm of satiating fibre. It also delivers vitamin C, potassium and vitamin B6 (essential for the formation of virtually all new cells in the body) and some phosphorous too, which is an essential nutrient for our bones. The fact is that this humble food is not just 'all carbs' as popularly thought; it also delivers many healthy nutrients.

## Your Heart's Friend

Potatoes are actually great for your heart too. They are high in magnesium and potassium—a powerful pair that together helps lower blood pressure. Also, the ratio of potassium (more) to sodium (less) in potatoes is just right. They have potent blood pressure-lowering compounds called kukoamines. Other known and good sources are a Chinese herb and goji berry, so obviously potatoes are easier to plate.

## High Antioxidant Count (Surprise!)

This will surprise you, but the antioxidant count (the value of oxygen radical absorbance capacity, or ORAC) for potatoes is fairly high, which means they help keep free radical damage (origin for most lifestyle disorders) down in the body. In fact, some reports suggest that phytochemicals in potatoes rival the amounts found in broccoli. Who would have thought!

### Did You Know?
It's best to have potatoes with the skin intact as without the jacket, the fibre content gets limited. Besides, the skin also has many nutrients—fibre, potassium, iron, calcium, zinc, phosphorus and B vitamins.

## Don't Fear It

Finally, the two big negatives thrown at potatoes—high in glycemic index (so, a blood sugar-raiser), and full of starch—don't hold much water. First, the glycemic index of potato has most likely been ranked incorrectly; the jury is still out on this. The glycemic index also depends on how we eat potatoes. When we have them cold (boiled and cooled), their glycemic index becomes lower. So, a cool potato salad is a fab way to enjoy this food. Also, potato is a brilliant source of resistant starch, which again is proving to be a big boon for our gut health.

## There's More...

You can drink potato water to cleanse your intestines and reduce the amount of acid in the gastrointestinal system. Just wash and dice a large potato, steep it overnight in one cup of water and add a pinch of sea salt. Strain and drink the water every morning on an empty stomach.

So, the bottom line is that you *can* eat potatoes without guilt, because as it turns out, it is in fact quite good for you.

## Easy Tips to Eat Potatoes

Few, quick serving ideas:

Purée roasted garlic, cooked potatoes and olive oil together to make delicious garlic mashed potatoes. Season to taste.

Toss steamed, diced potatoes with olive oil and fresh herbs of your choice.

Boil till tender and top with fresh dill.

Make aloo tikki on a nonstick pan and relish with mint chutney.

Bake and top with broccoli and cheese.

Mash and blend with low-fat milk.

Mix with cottage cheese or salsa, 2 tbsp beans and corn, and a dollop of sour cream for a Mexican lunch.

Try a potato au naturel or with your favourite healthy low-fat topping.

## At a Glance

The benefits of eating potatoes include,

- ❦ Scoring antioxidants and cutting free radicals to size
- ❦ Comfort food
- ❦ Strengthening your gut
- ❦ Lowering the blood pressure
- ❦ Boosting bone health

### Fun Fact
Potatoes have been around for a while now.
The traces of their presence dating back to
500 BCE have been found in the ancient ruins
of Peru and Chile.

Chapter 31

# PUMPKIN

### Not Just for Halloween

I fell in love with the ubiquitous pumpkin (kaddu) again when I experienced Halloween first-hand during my trip many years back to the city of Jackson in California. That sleepy town was awash with Halloween decorations, and trust me, they were all beyond brilliant. But what is still fresh in my mind is the interesting decorations made with whole pumpkins. Of course, one has heard and read enough about it, and seen pictures by the dozens, but only when you see the pumpkins so beautifully carved and all lighted—and so many of them together—that you realize it's really Halloween.

It was there that I heard the story of how it all began. Apparently the name 'jack-o'-lantern' comes from an Irish folk tale about a man named Stingy Jack, who was not allowed to enter either heaven or hell after his death, and was doomed to roam the Earth with a burning coal in a carved-out turnip. So, lights were placed inside turnips and potatoes with creepy faces carved into them to ward off evil spirits like Stingy Jack away. When immigrants from Ireland came to North America, they discovered that pumpkins—a fruit native to America—made for great lanterns.

Moreover, they also started incorporating pumpkins into their diet in many interesting ways and enjoyed this humble vegetable as one really should: as pumpkin lattes, pumpkin donuts, baked pumpkin fries, pumpkin risotto, and quinoa-stuffed pumpkin (believe you me!). It also showed up in everything from muffins to Greek yoghurts to cookies, and was even served mixed with granola for breakfast!

Now, we don't really celebrate Halloween in India, but that doesn't mean we can't have fun with pumpkin, because I believe this vegetable is straight out of a health fairy tale. In fact, this humble fruit (though it's considered a 'vegetable' in India) has been a huge part of Indian cuisine since forever, and is usually served after a puja is done at home. Till not so long back, it was a part of our regular menus too, but is mostly forgotten now.

### The Payback

Pumpkins were once recommended for removing freckles and curing snakebites. While the jury is still out on these uses, there is a lot going for this unusually shaped fruit that is part of the gourd family—of cucumbers, melons, cantaloupe and zucchini. For starters, it is 90 per cent water, extremely low calorie (just 26 gm calories per 100 gm pumpkin), and is loaded with fibre, which keeps your gut happy. Its brilliant orange colour comes from its ample supply of beta-carotene. This is converted to vitamin A in the body, which keeps our eyes sharp by protecting the cornea—the surface of the eye—and allows us to see under conditions of low light. Also, it is the best source of lutein and zeaxanthin, two crucial eye health compounds.

### Look Young

Eating pumpkin can help you look younger as the beta-carotene in it works as a natural sunblock and helps protect from the sun's wrinkle-causing UV rays. Carotenoids are effective wrinkle-fighting plant pigments that help neutralize free radicals in the skin (thus, delaying skin ageing). Pumpkin is also filled with powerful enzymes that help to cleanse the skin, and delay the degeneration of our body. It also delivers lots of potassium, an important electrolyte that keeps our muscles functioning at their best.

**The Vitamin C Advantage**

Pumpkin delivers vitamin C, which is essential for healthy skin as our body needs this vitamin to make collagen, a protein that keeps the skin strong and healthy. Vitamin C that is great for our immune system, especially in cold weather. It also reduces the risk of cataracts and macular degeneration—two of the leading causes of adult blindness.

**Antioxidant Advantage**

Your heart loves pumpkin as much as your taste buds do. That's because it is high in antioxidants, which neutralize free radicals, thus stopping them from damaging our cells, and also help protect LDL 'bad' cholesterol from oxidizing. When LDL cholesterol particles oxidize, they can clump together along the walls of blood vessels, which can restrict your vessels and raise your risk of heart diseases. Vitamins A and C together work as a kind of cell-defence squad, and shield the cells against cancer.

**If You Smoke...**

Pumpkin is loaded with a carotenoid called beta-cryptoxanthin, which gets converted to vitamin A in the body and helps substantially decrease the risk of lung cancer in smokers. It offers another plus: Smokers are usually low in vitamin C, which helps fend off free radicals that damage healthy lung cells, and this yellow goodness is loaded with it.

## Don't Throw the Seeds

If you have the habit of throwing out the seeds, you must know this: Pumpkin seeds pack a big punch too! They are rich in phytosterols, which help reduce LDL cholesterol, and tryptophan, which can keep our mood upbeat.

> **Did You Know?**
> Pumpkin flower is a good source of folate vitamins C and A, and tastes great mixed in salads and soups, sautéd or cheese-stuffed and batter-fried.

## Easy Tips to Eat Pumpkins

You could of course have some pumpkin subzi for lunch, or maybe pumpkin soup at night! Or maybe just to spice things up, try out some new dishes with this extremely versatile vegetable (risotto, latte, etc.). Add pumpkin to smoothies, purée into soups, mix into oats, stir into plain yoghurt and top with cinnamon, or whisk into cheesy pasta sauces.

Also try steaming pumpkin cubes and then dressing them with olive oil, ginger juliennes and pumpkin seeds.

Have a sweet tooth? Try pumpkin halwa. Also, check the recipe of pumpkin bread in the final section of this book; I had it in a small cafe in California and got the recipe from the chef there. It turned out fabulous! I have also included a recipe for pumpkin chips in the recipes section.

## At a Glance

The benefits of eating pumpkin include,

- Warding off cold and flu
- Keeping the eyes healthy and sharp
- Younger-looking skin
- Hydrating the body
- Losing weight easily

### Fun Fact

Pumpkins are grown on all but one continent (Antarctica) in the world.

Chapter 32

# RADISH

### Dish Up the Radish

When my mother is staying with us, the menu automatically changes for the better. Suddenly, all the healthy, forgotten dishes start getting cooked. The regular dishes—dal chawal and those same two or three subzis cooked by rotation get replaced by interesting, super-healthy, and sometimes slightly unusual dishes. And the best news is that radish (mooli) makes an appearance on our plates more often. For example, mooli ka parantha wolfed down with dhania-amla-mint chutney and beaten curd, and my childhood favourite mooli bhurjee with the leaves, relished with missi roti...and more such dishes. I don't know anyone else (like my mom) who can eat radishes with so much joy! She *loves* them! And thankfully that seems to have passed on to me too.

### Nutrition Punch

A winter staple, radish is very good for us. This slightly bitter root is amazingly low in calories (100 gm of radish gives less than 20 calories), is loaded with vitamin C, and is rich in folate, vitamin B6, riboflavin, thiamin and minerals like iron, magnesium and copper.

### A Weight Watcher's Friend

Radish is high in roughage, contains a lot of water, and is low on the glycemic index too (keeps blood sugar stable), so it is a great food even for those who are watching their weight or sugar levels.

## Antioxidants Ahoy!

Radish is a great source of anthocyanins, a type of antioxidant that is great for our heart and displays anti-cancer and anti-inflammatory properties. In fact, the folic acid, vitamin C and anthocyanins in radish make it a very effective cancer-fighting food.

## Heart-friendly

Eating radishes regularly keeps cholesterol levels in check, and the potassium in it keeps blood pressure low.

> **Did You Know?**
> Have you been eating a lot of junk food and getting too tipsy of late? Eat some radishes to cleanse the blood and raise oxygen level. It's your easy ticket to a natural detox.

## Your Cold Weather Friend

Radish is fabulous for winter months as it naturally decreases the congestion of the respiratory system, cuts the irritation of the nose, throat and windpipe, and decongests the lungs—symptoms that accompany frequent colds, infections, allergies and other causes common during these months. So, a mooli parantha or a radish salad, when in season, is undoubtedly a no-brainer to keep winter ailments in check.

## Eat the Leaves too

Why radish leaves, you ask? That's because the leaves are even more nutrient-dense than the radish. They deliver lots of iron, which helps cut fatigue, prevent anaemia and boost the haemoglobin level. They are a good source of vitamin C (as much as six times more per serving than the radish itself), which boosts immunity big time and delivers some vitamin A, thiamine (vitamin B1), pyridoxin (vitamin B6), folic acid (vitamin B9), calcium and the hard-to-find phosphorus, potassium and magnesium. In fact, the high level of potassium, iron, vitamin C and dietary fibre found in radish greens help strengthen the heart and keep our cholesterol levels sorted.

### Anti-ageing

Radish greens display an impressive antioxidant capacity too, ranking right up there with other big shots like broccoli and kale. This means that they can help fight against oxidative stress and chronic diseases in the body. They, in fact, have some unique antioxidants called sulforaphane indoles and anthocyanins, which are known for their cancer-prevention abilities. Having enough antioxidants in the diet is actually great news for our skin too, as they help the skin to stay young and also reduce the appearance of blemishes and scars.

### Beat Bloating

The best news though is that radish leaves are a natural diuretic—perfect for those who suffer from water retention and feel bloated all the time. The vitamin B6 in them even helps dissolve kidney stones and improves liver function.

### Prevent Constipation

These leaves also demonstrate strong laxative properties as they stimulate peristaltic motion and prevent a number of gastrointestinal problems. Thus, they naturally help ease constipation and a bloated stomach, and keep our gut smiling by improving its nutrient-absorption efficiency.

**The Rad Root**

Radish is high in fibre (100 gm radish gives a whopping 4 gm fibre), so it helps you feel—and stay—full for longer. This will help you keep a check on your cravings between meals and curb overeating. It is high in fibre, and has a low glycemic index, so it's a fabulous food for diabetics too and helps keep blood sugar level under control.

**Easy Tips to Eat Radishes**

Make one radish part of your salad every day. In fact, if you need some crunch in your salads but want to keep it healthy, add radishes instead of croutons. Cook mooli subzi, or use radishes to make sambar and chutney like they do in the southern part of our country. You can even pickle and eat them with your regular meals, or roast them with garlic and add to pastas, sandwiches and salads.

Try this salad: In a salad bowl, combine sliced radishes and cucumbers, and chopped green onions. To make the dressing, whisk together equal parts yoghurt, sour cream, chopped garlic, a little bit of olive oil, and salt and pepper to taste in a mixing bowl. Add the dressing to the salad; mix well, chill and enjoy.

Also never throw the leaves—cook them with some radish (or carrot) pieces in mustard oil with just salt, asafoetida, carom seeds, ginger and green chillies. You can also add them to salads, sandwiches and dals. You can even make a side dish by just wilting them and adding some butter and lemon juice, or mix them up with potatoes and onions and make a nice soup. Or try a radish green pesto (my favourite): Mix some radish leaves with freshly grated parmesan cheese, garlic, olive oil, almonds and walnuts (or sunflower seeds). Spread over a cracker or a toast and have it.

The peppery, earthy taste of radish and its leaves takes a little getting used to, but it's totally worth the benefits.

### At a Glance

The benefits of eating radish include,

- Acting as a natural detox
- Keeping your blood pressure tamed
- Easing constipation and a bloated stomach
- Reducing blemishes and scars
- Preventing winter congestion

### Fun Fact
Radish was so highly regarded in ancient Greece that its gold replicas were presented to their god, Apollo.

Mini Chapter VIII

## POLLUTION ANTIDOTES

**Fixit Tip 83:** The antihistamines in mint leaves are perfect antidotes for pollution. Eat mint chutney with every meal, and add mint to your stir-fries liberally.

**Fixit Tip 84:** Begin your day with ginger tea and have a cup when you get back home after work. It helps remove pollutants from the air passages before they reach the lungs.

**Fixit Tip 85:** Clove is an expectorant that helps to break up phlegm in the throat, and keeps respiratory tract infections away. Drink clove tea and place one under your tongue (and keep sucking on it slowly) whenever you step out in the pollution.

**Fixit Tip 86:** Drink 10-15 ml of tulsi juice to clear pollutants from the respiratory tract.

**Fixit Tip 87:** The resveratrol in grapes helps cut the inflammation of the lungs due to pollution and keep the lungs fighting fit.

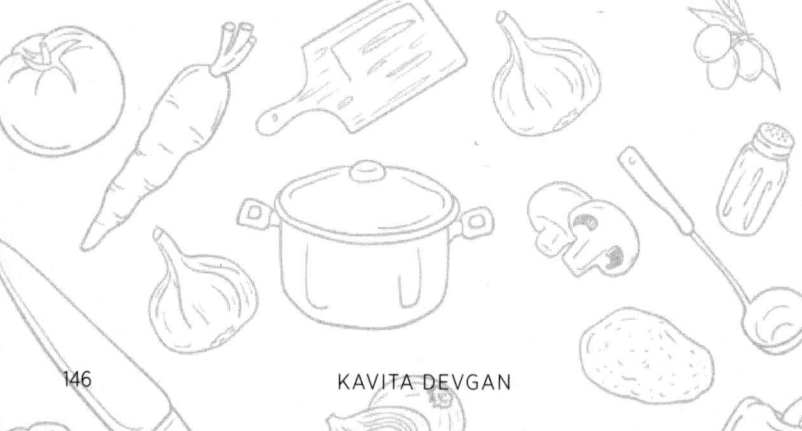

Chapter 33

# SATTU

## Quintessentially Indian

In ancient India, people were aware of how good sattu (roasted gram flour) is, and that is why it was eaten every day (and still is in the hinterlands of Punjab, Madhya Pradesh, Telangana, Uttar Pradesh, Rajasthan and the eastern states of India). Today's generation though has decided to simply ignore it, as most tag it a poor man's protein. That's not right!

In fact, I don't get it—protein is protein. And when we are struggling to score enough protein, it is a defeatist attitude to ignore this power-packed inexpensive instant food (India's oldest I think), which is so easily available. We need a marketing blitz to make it cool and also package it attractively to sell it to the youth.

I feel spreading information about it might also open some eyes and minds and bring it back on our plates.

## A Super-superfood

Sattu provides instant energy, and is a brilliant source of good quality vegetarian protein (100 gm of sattu delivers close to 20 gm of protein). It has a lot of fibre (close to 22 gm), most of which is insoluble fibre, which is great for our gut and helps cleanse the stomach and detox the body. It is a wonderfood for those who are suffering from gas, acidity and constipation.

## Safe for Everyone

Sattu is low on the glycemic index (the glycemic index ranks foods on how they affect our blood sugar levels), so it is good for diabetics, and being low in sodium, it's safe for people suffering from hypertension too. It also has calcium (yes, it's good for our bones), iron, manganese, magnesium and vitamins C and A.

### Did You Know?
Sattu is a natural coolant. so it's a perfect antidote to the sweltering summertime heat.

## It Is Calorific, Though

Two tbsp (25 gm) of sattu will give you 100 calories, which is a little steep, but acceptable when you consider the benefits it delivers (5 gm of protein and fibre each). Another big benefit is that it doesn't get spoilt for a really long time.

Sattu is an indigenous, completely natural and safe protein powder, which delivers health and helps us lose weight. Also, it's incredibly delicious.

## Easy Tips to Eat Sattu

Traditionally, sattu has always been made with chana dal, by dry roasting them in sand (like peanuts), sieving and then pounding to a powder, but some people now add some chickpeas too for a twist in flavour. In Punjab though, barley (jau) sattu is more popular. Now of course, all kinds of sattu powders are easily available commercially.

Sattu is quite versatile and can be consumed in multiple ways. Sattu sherbat, either sweet (with jaggery) or savoury (with salt and roasted cumin powder) is very popular. You can also add some lemon juice and mint leaves. It is an instant energy drink and I personally love to pair it with another superfood—coconut water—to further boost its electrolyte content, or with buttermilk to boost protein even further.

Sattu is eaten too. Some options are the famous litti of Bihar and Jharkhand, sattu-stuffed roti/paratha, upma and ladoo. Take my advice and pair sattu parantha with your subzis, and also try sattu and onion pakoras. You'll thank me! Sattu can even be mixed with sugar and water (or a pickle), and had for breakfast, which'll keep hunger pangs and cravings away till lunchtime. Also, if sattu is had regularly, it will build muscle mass effectively, which is great for growing children.

## At a Glance

The benefits of eating sattu include,

- Deriving superlative protein
- Getting instant energy
- Staying cool in the summers
- Cleansing the stomach
- Scoring calcium and other minerals

### Fun Fact
According to Maharashtrian folklore, sattu was a favourite food of King Shivaji when he was engaged in full-scale guerrilla warfare against the Mughals and their allies.

Chapter 34

# SPINACH

### The Spinach Story

Not many people know that spinach actually became famous because of a decimal point mistake. In 1870, German chemist Erich von Wolf, while researching the amount of iron in spinach and other green vegetables, wrote 35 mg iron in a 100 gm serving of spinach by mistake (when actually the correct value is 3.5 mg). This missed decimal point and thereafter, Popeye's much-publicized love for spinach made it the flavour of the times, and helped increase its consumption. This myth is known as 'SPIDES'–Spinach Popeye Iron Decimal Error Story.

Even though Wolf's error was corrected in 1937, the spinach-iron myth continues till today. I still hear a lot of mothers telling their children to eat spinach for its iron content. The truth is that due to the presence of a high level of oxalate, which inhibits iron absorption, most of the iron found in spinach is of no use to the body (though, boiling helps neutralize the oxalates to a large extent). In fact, foods like beans and tofu are better foods to eat for scoring iron.

### Nutrient Load

Lack of absorbable iron notwithstanding, this leafy vegetable is still a wonderfood. Spinach has a dozen anti-cancer agents and also a huge antioxidant repertoire. It is rich in vitamin A and delivers two of the carotenoids–lutein and zeaxanthin—in abundance, both of which are great for our vision.

## Super-strong Bones

Spinach may not have provided iron to Popeye, but it did make him strong by gifting him strong bones. It is the richest source of vitamin K after kale. The vitamin K1 in it prevents the functioning of osteoclasts (the cells that break down bones) and it forms vitamin K2 in the intestines (thanks to the friendly bacteria), which helps anchor calcium molecules inside the bone. Besides vitamin K, spinach also has good amounts of calcium and magnesium, other bone-supportive nutrients.

## Talking of Magnesium...

In fact, 250 gm of spinach will deliver 200 mg of magnesium, which is half of our daily requirement of 400 mg. Enough magnesium helps prevent muscle cramps, facial and eye tics, poor sleep, hyperactivity, constipation, frequent headaches and restless legs syndrome.

## Brain Food

A healthy magnesium level provides protection against depression, as it is important for the release and binding of adequate amounts of serotonin—the happy hormone—in the brain. Spinach also delivers lots of vitamin B6, which is important for our memory preservation.

> **Did You Know?**
> Spinach is both a diuretic (facilitates removal of excess water from the body) and a laxative (helps in the emptying of bowels).

### Your Waist Shrinker

Thylakoids in spinach promote the release of satiety hormones and thus help cut cravings and deliver weight loss. It also reduces levels of ghrelin, the hunger hormone. So, a serving of spinach with your meal may actually help you feel full, helping you avoid the temptation to tuck into something sinful.

### Your Heart's Friend

Thanks to the nitrate content in spinach, it helps keep your heart smiling. Up until recently, nitrate wasn't thought to have any nutritional value at all. It was even being suggested that it might be toxic. But now it is clear that nitrates found in a plateful of spinach help open up our blood vessels to lower blood pressure, and also make our muscles more efficient during a workout.

Eating more spinach can also help lower our homocysteine (a major risk factor for heart disease) level by increasing the amount of folate (a B vitamin) we get through our diet. In fact, lower levels of homocysteine have been linked to reducing the risk of heart disease, osteoporosis, bone fractures and dementia.

### The Alkaline Advantage

Our diet these days is primarily acidic (highly processed and packaged foods), which leads to higher toxic residue in the body (which means, more fatigue and lifestyle diseases), so eating primarily alkaline foods is the way to go. And spinach is one of the top five alkaline foods around (other four are: eggplant, cucumber, watermelon and lemon).

## Easy Tips to Eat Spinach

This nutrient-dense vegetable seems humble, but its versatility as a salad base, a smoothie add-in, or a superfood side-dish is unbelievable. There's a way to cook spinach right. Don't overcook it; instead just boil it uncovered for 1 minute to leach out oxalic acid, which interferes with the absorption of some nutrients.

I love to eat it like this: Stir-fry boiled spinach in olive oil for a minute, then season with salt and pepper, add a pinch of nutmeg, and finally stir in some feta cheese. It is amazingly delicious.

You could juice it too. This way the beta-carotene stored in its cell membranes becomes even easier for the body to absorb.

A green smoothie (spinach with pineapple and ginger) for breakfast is a great idea. I also love this simple smoothie: Blend a handful of spinach leaves, 1 cucumber, ½ green apple and 1 cup fresh coconut milk. You can also add some seeds for a dose of good fat.

Or make a salad: Mix baby spinach, and chopped oranges and mushrooms. Add a dressing made of honey, apple cider vinegar, olive oil, a pinch of salt and some poppy seeds. Toss and eat.

And try adding boiled spinach to rice; it tastes fabulous.

## At a Glance

The benefits of eating spinach include,

- Providing vitamin A (carotenoids) for our eyes
- Supporting our bone health
- Detoxifying the body

- Helping lower blood pressure
- Helping us stay happier and boosting our memory

**Fun Fact**
Spinach is 90 per cent water!
You can watch it shrink as it cooks.

Chapter 35

# SWEET LIME

### Not Just a Fruit for when You Are Unwell

Very often we keep talking about oranges and lemons, but one citrus fruit that does not get much press is the sweet lime (mosambi). Not much is known about it, and I don't see too many fruit carts laden with this fruit anymore, unlike say oranges or even kinnows. In fact, its origin is misunderstood too. Most think that it originated in Indonesia and China, but it most likely originated in the hills of Meghalaya and Nagaland. There is no clear verdict on this, but what we do know is that there are umpteen benefits of consuming this fruit and its juice—and that it is not just a fruit to be had when one is sick!

### Beats Dehydration

Mosambi is an extremely hydrating food, as it not only quenches your thirst, but also provides you essential minerals and vitamins that reduce the risk associated with dehydration.

### Your Weight Loss Friend

One medium-sized mosambi gives you only about 60–70 calories and keeps you satisfied for long, thanks to its high water and fibre content. Its high citric acid level curbs hunger pangs, and boosts our metabolism, making it a perfect food to turn to when we are trying to lose weight.

It is best to eat the fruit whole, but if you are opting for the juice, please don't strain it, so you can score the fibrous pulp and stay full for longer. The pulp will also keep the bowel healthy and prevent constipation.

## Lots of Nutrients

Mosambi is a rich source of vitamin C (ascorbic acid), which helps build strong immunity. Besides, we need a daily supply of this water-soluble vitamin as we cannot store it in our body, and mosambi does the deed well. It also delivers lots of potassium and some vitamin B, copper, calcium, iron and phosphorus. It also contains folic acid, which helps to strengthen our bones and joints. Thanks to the high electrolyte (particularly potassium) content, mosambi helps reduce muscle cramps and is a perfect food to hydrate the body after a rigorous workout.

> **Did You Know?**
> Sweet lime is packed with antioxidants that help reduce inflammation, regulate the immune system and increase resistance to infections, particularly colds.

## A Brilliant Cleanser

Mosambi juice acts as a potent detoxifying agent as it helps flush out toxins and thus neutralize the harmful effects of junk food (which most of us are guilty of consuming), stress and pollution.

It contains limonenes, a family of chemicals that benefits our health. D-limonene works as an anti-inflammatory agent and fights cancer growth (by promoting the death of cancer cells).

## In Sickness and in Health

It's true that mosambi actually helps when you are unwell more than any other citrus fruit. It scores over other citrus fruits because it has a mild and palatable flavour, which people prefer when they are sick. Oranges and lemons can taste sour, but mosambi tastes sweet, and that is why a lot of people prefer it.

It is less acidic compared to oranges and lemons, which helps reduce stomach acidity and makes it alkaline, thus helping to heal the painful peptic ulcers or sores that may develop along the lining of your stomach, upper intestine and the lining of your esophagus, especially when one has gastro issues.

When we are sick, our taste buds and digestion go on a holiday. Here, mosambi helps stimulate the salivary glands to secrete enzymes that ease digestion. Its high amount of potassium also helps combat diarrhoea, which often accompanies infections, or is a side effect of strong medicines.

Potassium helps prevent and treat dehydration too, another common side effect when we are sick.

Mosambi is great for our liver as well, as it boosts its fuctioning and helps combat jaundice symptoms, like fever and vomiting.

## Easy Tips to Eat Sweet Limes

So, eat sweet lime peeled and raw as a snack, cook it and preserve it as a jam, or eat it in a salad. Have more of it every day when in season, not just when you are sick!

They even taste great in desserts—their zesty, mildly acidic flavour can add a great balance to sweet notes, making desserts taste lighter and more refreshing. So add it to cakes, pies, sorbets, puddings, etc.

## At a Glance

The benefits of eating mosambi include,

- Preventing dehydration
- Recovering faster from an illness
- Making the stomach alkaline
- Boosting inflammation
- Strengthening the bones and joints

### Fun Fact

British sailors in the nineteenth century often suffered from scurvy, a disease that results from vitamin C deficiency. But because lemons were not widely available and thus expensive, these sailors were told to have one lime every day to prevent this disease. This is why today this generation of sailors are known as 'limeys'.

Chapter 36

# SWEET POTATO

## Really Sweet Sweet Potatoes

Sweet potatoes just get the rap because they belong to the root family (which also includes potatoes). These underappreciated tubers actually have a lot going for them nutritionally, and are packed with unbelievable goodness. While staying at a wellness resort near Pune, I had sweet potato cooked interestingly in two meals in a row: sweet potato-stuffed parantha for breakfast, and then as a side (mashed and mixed with zucchini) for a grilled dish. Both were so delicious that it made me wonder why we don't use them more often in cooking, or rather why we simply don't eat these powerhouse root vegetables more.

## Nutrition Punch

Sweet potatoes deliver a good amount of vitamin C, which helps boost immunity, and two essential nutrients for heart health: potassium and magnesium. They are loaded with essential B vitamins—niacin (B3), pantothenic acid (B5) and pyridoxine (B6s). Its B5 aids in weight loss, supports healthy hair and skin and helps lower cholesterol, and B6 is important for brain function and development. It is also involved in the process of making serotonin and norepinephrine, which are chemicals that transmit signals in the brain. Niacin regulates digestion, improves the cholesterol level, is great for our skin and also for maintaining the mobility of our joints, which helps keep arthritis at bay.

## Eye Tonic

Sweet potatoes are a natural source of beta-carotene, which gets converted into vitamin A in the body. In fact, you need to eat just one medium sweet potato to score your daily requirement of vitamin A. The bonus is that the beta-carotene they provide is better absorbed than what we get from green leafy vegetables. Tip: Always include some fat in your sweet potato dishes (some nuts, seeds or a drizzle of cold-pressed oil) as it significantly increases the absorption of beta-carotene from sweet potatoes.

## Antioxidants Ahoy!

This humble food has antioxidant properties (vitamins A, C and E), which help in preventing oxidative damage and thus help keep most lifestyle diseases like cardiac disorders, diabetes, etc. away. In fact, beta-carotene is a powerful antioxidant that helps ward off cancer and protects against the effects of ageing. In addition, sweet potatoes are rich in anthocyanin, which is a pigment that keeps inflammation in the body in check.

## Cleanser and Beauty Aid

Both vitamin A and anthocyanins also help boost liver function, which in turn helps boost weight loss and keep harmful cholesterol in the body in check. Beta-carotene also helps protect the cells from sun damage, prevents the ageing of the skin, and naturally exfoliates it too.

## Fibre Load

Sweet potatoes contain more fibre than potatoes. For example, 250 gm of sweet potatoes will deliver about 200 calories and 7.5 gm of fibre, whereas a similar amount of potato will deliver similar calories and about 5 gm of fibre. In fact, it is a great constipation-relieving food due to its high resistant starch content, which functions like soluble, fermentable fibre, reaching the intestines and helping boost the good bacteria.

> **Did You Know?**
> Sweet potato is an excellent antacid and it's great for people who suffer from acidity frequently.

## Safe for Everyone

Sweet potatoes are naturally sweet, but they have a lower glycemic index than potatoes, so the natural sugars are slowly released into the bloodstream and don't cause a sharp spike in blood sugar. Also, eating sweet potatoes can significantly increase the level of adiponectin (a protein) in the blood, which actually helps regulate the insulin metabolism better. Thus, they are good for diabetics when eaten in moderation. When you add it to a meal and pair it with some protein, it will help keep you full longer.

## Sleep Like a Baby

Sweet potatoes are a sleeper's dream as not only do they provide sleep-inducing complex carbohydrates, but also contain the muscle-relaxant potassium.

## Easy Tips to Eat Sweet Potatoes

Sweet potatoes are very versatile. The best ways to cook them are steaming or roasting, but they can also be boiled and pureed to be used as porridge. My personal favourite: The street-side, spicy, lemony sharkarkandi chaat. Or try this: Bake sweet potato with 1 tsp of olive oil, a dash of cinnamon and a sprinkle of black salt.

## At a Glance

The benefits of eating sweet potatoes include,

- Saving your eyes
- Preventing acidity
- Keeping your skin younger-looking
- Preventing constipation
- Keeping you full longer

### Fun Fact
One of the oldest vegetables known to man, sweet potato relics dating back 10,000 years have been discovered in Peruvian caves.

## Mini Chapter IX

### LOSE IT

**Fixit Tip 88:** Are you craving sugar? Try this almond treat. Have an almond stacked on top of a dried apricot. It tastes better than a cookie.

**Fixit Tip 89:** Pine nuts contain pinolenic acid, which triggers the release of an appetite-suppressing hormone cholecystokinin (CCK), and so they are a good weight-loss aid. They also pack in a lot of heart-healthy fatty acids that not just quell hunger hormones and provide satiety, but also boost the metabolism and burn belly fat (the most dangerous for our health).

**Fixit Tip 90:** The complex carbohydrates-and-fibre combination of yams (5 gm in one cup) releases energy gradually in the body, slowing the rate at which their sugars are released and absorbed into the bloodstream—a perfect food if you are looking at losing some weight. Just munch on them, add to a salad or roast thin slices and relish with some chutney.

**Fixit Tip 91:** Eat foods that take more time to prepare. This way you'll eat less of the very same foods. Always buy unshelled peanuts and pistachios rather than salted, shelled ones.

**Fixit Tip 92:** Here's the best weight-loss tip ever—place fruits like peaches, plums, grapes, apples, pears, bananas, oranges and sweet limes in a bowl on the dining table. That's how you'll reach for them when you are hungry.

**Fixit Tip 93**: Blend 2 cups of papaya with a pinch of cardamom and salt each. To this, add ½ tsp lime juice and 1 tbsp soaked (for 2 hours) sabja seeds. This is a perfect antidote to your cravings.

**Fixit Tip 94:** Are cravings troubling you? Begin your day with lemon juice in warm water plus a pinch of cinnamon. This drink will increase your metabolic rate, make the body alkaline and keep blood sugar stable.

Chapter 37

# WALNUT

## A Superstar Nut

This superstar nut is perfect for your entire family. Add its crunch daily to your family's diet. 1 ounce (14 halves) of walnuts provides 4 gm protein, 2 gm fibre, lots of manganese, magnesium, phosphorus, zinc, selenium, some vitamin B and loads of E. And the fats it has—MUFA and Omega-3—are all 'good' fats. It is calorie-dense though (an ounce gives 180 calories), so watch your portions. The trick is to replace the 'saturated fat' calories with the high-quality beneficial fat that walnuts provide.

## Antioxidants Galore

Yes, walnut has the strongest line-up of antioxidants (vitamin E, ellagic acid, melatonin and carotenoids) amongst all the nuts. They are second only to blackberries. In fact, one study even proved that a handful of walnuts (802 mg) has significantly more phenolics (antioxidants) than a glass of apple juice (117 mg), a milk chocolate bar (205 mg), and a glass of red wine (372 mg).

## Brain Food

It is the ultimate brain food—the Omega-3 present in walnuts help the brain fluid to function properly and also help beat depression, attention-deficit hyperactivity disorder (ADHD), and Alzheimer's disease (vitamin E arrests age-related cognitive decline). Walnuts are also great for ensuring adequate shut-eye and to buff up the memory. That is why I ask mothers to begin giving their children walnuts (crushed/mashed and added to their cereals) from the time they are six months old to help in the development of their brain.

## Save Your Heart

The E in walnuts is in a form that is very heart-protective (gamma-tocopherol), and its Omega-3 helps lower cholesterol levels, reduce inflammation and improve blood flow through the arteries.

## Sugar Buster

Walnuts protect the body against diabetes as well. The good fats and magnesium in walnuts do the deed. And you need only 4 halves a day to get this protection, which is not difficult at all.

> **Did You Know?**
> Have trouble sleeping? Just pop in a few halves of walnuts regularly before bedtime as this will boost the production of melatonin, a hormone that regulates sleep.

## Prevent Depression

People with a significant level of depression also suffer from a low level of docosahexaenoic and eicosapentanoic acids, which can be replenished easily via walnuts.

## Making Babies

Chomping on walnuts helps boost sperm count and motility. What is it that does the trick? Possibly, the Omega-3 in it and also the folic acid, zinc and selenium that walnuts are loaded with.

### Did You Know?
Walnuts can be eaten directly from the tree, but the flavour is milder and the texture is softer compared to nuts that have been dried.

## Easy Tips to Eat Walnuts

Walnuts are a wonderful snack, but I say, begin your day with them—just pop a few in, or dice and add to your cereals and fruit salads. Or like me, team them with a few raisins or anjeer—to make a delightful chewy dessert after a meal. The bittersweet combination is brilliant!

Want to try something new? Make a pesto sauce with a twist: Use walnuts instead of pine nuts and mix them with olive oil, garlic, salt and fresh basil using a mortar and pestle. It's delicious!

## At a Glance

The benefits of eating walnuts include,

- Keeping your brain and memory sharp
- Preventing diabetes
- Scoring inflammation-cutting Omega-3
- Preventing depression
- Saving your heart
- Boosting fertility

**Fun Fact**

Have you noticed how the walnut shell looks like a human skull and the nut itself looks like a brain? This is why walnuts were called 'karyon'—meaning 'head'—by the ancient Greeks!

Chapter 38

# WATER CHESTNUT

## The Underrated Singhara

When I was growing up, water chestnuts, called singharas (or shinghodas) in north India, were very often our family's default snack for car journeys when they were in season. I still remember how much fun my sister and I had chomping on these juicy heart-shaped delights, and by the time we would go through the lot we had bought, most journeys would be almost over. It was a tedious task, the peeling and eating, but no one complained as it was always fun.

Unfortunately, even though I have spotted singharas on carts every now and then, I somehow did not eat them for a couple of decades, waylaid by other, more interesting snack options available. But that was only till I made a serious, conscious effort to get singharas—also called paani-phal (water fruit)—back in my diet a couple of years ago and began eating them happily again. I realized then how much I had missed their mild, sweet taste and crisp, crunchy texture.

## Nutrient Powerhouse

Singharas are really good for us; we must eat more of them because, not only are they just super-delish, but are a powerhouse of nutrients too.

The first benefit is that they are fat-, cholesterol- and gluten-free, and have a very low level of sodium and calories (100 gm give just 90 calories; one water chestnut is approximately 9 calories) and a decent amount of fibre too. Tell me, how many snacks can offer all this?

They are an excellent source of potassium, a mineral that is essential for proper functioning of the muscles and nerves and also helps bust water retention and lower blood pressure by balancing sodium. They also deliver bone-strengthening calcium and other minerals like iodine and manganese (which help in maintaining proper functioning of the thyroid gland) and copper, zinc, B vitamins and vitamin E, all of which are extremely essential for us to stay healthy.

## Almost Medicinal

Ayurvedic and Unani systems of medicines have recognized water chestnuts since forever for their medicinal benefits. They help quench thirst and are perfect to beat the scorching heat of summers, thanks to their excellent cooling properties. Apparently, they have neuroprotective properties too, and may reverse oxidative damage in the brain caused by ageing.

**Did You Know?**
Singharas are a great detoxifying agent and help flush out toxins from the body, and have antibacterial, antiviral, anti-cancer and antioxidant properties too.

## Easy Tips to Eat Water Chestnuts

While the best way to relish water chestnuts are in their raw, peeled form, they can even be steamed or lightly sautéed, and pair rather well with a few vegetables. The best part is that they don't lose their crunchiness on being cooked or canned and have been an integral part of Chinese cooking since ancient times.

We don't use them much in Indian cooking, except the singhara flour, which is commonly used during navratras, but maybe it's time to change that. I remember having an amazing pumpkin soup with water chestnuts, and a water chestnut and beetroot halwa at a resort near Pune and they both tasted delish.

I feel this is an interesting idea as incorporating water chestnuts in our cooking will not just make our everyday food more exciting, but also ensure a stockpile of essential trace minerals and vitamins for our body.

### At a Glance

The benefits of eating singhara include,

- Busting water retention
- Proper functioning of the muscles and nerves
- Detoxification of the body
- Loading up on multiple nutrients and fibre
- Improving thyroid function

**Fun Fact**
Singharas are actually a seed,
not a fruit or vegetable!

Chapter 39

# WATERMELON

### Wonderful Watermelon

On a hot summer day, what is the most refreshing fruit? Definitely watermelon (tarbooz)! It is one of summertime's essential fruits because with the heat wave on, this red delight is a perfect answer to cool you down and quench your thirst instantly as it is more than 90 per cent water. But there are many more reasons to bite into that crisp, juicy slice of watermelon—a fruit that can be traced back to Africa!

### Water Loaded

Staying properly hydrated is extremely important to stay safe from the ravages of the skyrocketing mercury, particularly during the summers. Although plain water and other beverages meet a significant amount of fluid requirements, watermelon is a perfect add-on. It is an easy (and tasty) way to give dehydration and related-summer problems a skip.

### Low in Calories, yet Filling

One cup of watermelon chunks (about 150 gm) give only 40 calories, but because of its high water content, it is filling. It is fat-free, low in calories, yet offers a great energy boost!

### It's A, B and C...

It is practically a multivitamin in itself. Vitamin A found in watermelon is important for optimal eye health, helps prevent night blindness, and boosts immunity by enhancing the infection-fighting actions of white blood cells (lymphocytes). Vitamin B6 found in watermelon is used by the body to manufacture brain chemicals (neurotransmitters)—serotonin, melatonin and dopamine—which help the body cope with anxiety and panic and keep one happy and calm. Vitamin C helps bolster the immune system against infections and viruses and can protect the body from harmful free radicals that can accelerate ageing and conditions like cataracts. Vitamin C is also required for the production and maintenance of collagen, boosting the body's ability to fight infection, and keep the capillaries and gums healthy. It also has lots of trace minerals (copper, iron, manganese, selenium and zinc).

### K Pop

Watermelon gets the 'heart healthy' seal of approval, because it is low in sodium and high in potassium (K), which helps regulate fluids and the mineral balance in the body, aids in muscle contraction, and helps transmit nerve impulses. A low potassium level can lead to muscle cramps, so sipping on watermelon juice can keep painful cramps at bay.

### Hypertension Buster

Watermelon's biggest plus is that it is the richest edible natural source of L-citrulline, which gets converted into L-arginine, an amino acid that is essential for the formation of nitric oxide. Nitric oxide, in turn, helps regulate blood pressure in the body and keeps it in the healthy range. L-arginine also helps improve blood flow and other aspects of our cardiac health. So, the easiest (and a tasty) way to keep the blood pressure down is to have this red delight.

### Stay Thin

Conversion of citrulline into arginine also helps prevent excess accumulation of fat in fat cells due to blocked activity of an enzyme called TNAP. And as easily as that, this can help you transform to a thinner you.

### Beating Cancer

Lycopene is what makes watermelons red (other sources include tomatoes, red and pink grapefruit, and guava). Look carefully at watermelon juice and you'll see little specks of red in it. That's lycopene. Lycopene, like vitamin C, neutralizes cell-damaging free radicals and helps prevent age-related diseases and even cancer.

**Did You Know?**
Drinking watermelon juice before a hard workout helps reduce heart rate and muscle soreness.

### Easy Tips to Eat Watermelons

In China, watermelon is stir-fried, stewed and often pickled and used as a vegetable. You don't just have to eat it like a cut fruit or as part of a salad, this versatile fruit allows you to get experimental with it too. Scoop out the fruit and cut the rind like a basket for an even prettier fruit salad. But there's more to watermelon than just slicing and juicing. You can try these ideas: Puree watermelon chunks, and then freeze into tasty pops.

You can also add watermelon balls to gelatine salads for fresh flavour and colour.

Freeze watermelon cubes or chunks to use as ice cubes in beverages.

To create a serving bowl, cut the watermelon lengthwise. Scoop out the flesh and combine with other fruits. Drain the empty watermelon shell before filling with the fruit mix.

Cut the flesh of the watermelon into festive shapes and top with cottage cheese. Or make a super summer salad with watermelon balls and chopped celery, topped with heavy whipped cream.

And next time, eat some part of the white rind too (cut the green layer carefully, leave some white portion in or scrape out the rind thinly and eat). That's because this is the most nutritious part of the fruit and has more vitamin A, B6, C, potassium and zinc than the red, juicy part.

## At a Glance

The benefits of eating watermelon include,

- Staying thin
- Hydrating the body
- Keeping blood pressure down
- Preventing muscle cramps
- Beating cancer

### Fun Fact
Egyptians grew watermelons some 5,000 years ago and they were held in such regard that their seeds and paintings were placed in the tombs of many Egyptian kings.

Chapter 40

# YOGHURT

### Eat Yoghurt to Save Your Life

I love milk, so it's a huge sore point with me that I am lactose intolerant and that's precisely why I can't resist mentioning it in every possible article. It's my way of whining and complaining. But the good news is that I can handle yoghurt well, so I turned to it to score enough calcium, and fell in love with it. Yoghurt, besides being a bonafide nutritional gold mine, is full of with beneficial bacteria that we *must* consume for our health.

Lactose intolerance is the inability to digest the primary carbohydrates in milk due to a deficiency of the enzyme, lactase, in the body. This deficiency results in gas, bloating, diarrhoea and other unpleasant gastrointestinal problems on consumption of milk. As lactose is already converted to lactic acid during the manufacture of yoghurt, it is more easily digested by people with lactose intolerance than other dairy products. So, for the millions of people who cannot tolerate milk products, yoghurt with live and active cultures is an easily digestible dairy source of calcium.

### Nutrition Punch

One cup (250 gm) of yoghurt gives about 150 calories and is loaded with protein and calcium. It is actually almost as good a source of potassium as a banana and an even better source of calcium and protein as compared to milk. A cup of yoghurt delivers 8–10 gm of protein. Plus it supplies protein that is complete and pre-digested. A cup of yoghurt also delivers a whopping 450 mg of calcium (compare that with 300 mg in a cup of milk—250 ml); this is 30 per cent to 40 per cent of most people's daily needs.

**Did You Know?**
Lactic acid in yoghurt aids protein, calcium and iron assimilation in the body.

### The B Benefit

Do you want to score enough B vitamins? Just have two servings of yoghurt every day. Yoghurt sets up an efficient little factory in the intestinal tract and manufactures B vitamins for you.

### Stomach Soother

Yoghurt kills bad 'bugs' in the body and helps maintain a healthy balance of intestinal bacteria. It also prevents and treats diarrhoea and other such ailments. In fact, it helps restore the digestive tract to its normal condition after a course of antibiotics. The drugs often wipe out every bacterium in their path, good and bad, altering the natural balance of the digestive tract. When harmful bacteria dominate the intestine, essential nutrients are not produced and the levels of damaging substances like carcinogens and toxins rise.

### Delays Ageing

Eating yoghurt can help delay the ageing process and prolong life. Bulgaria is known for the longevity of its people. Their secret? Bulgarians have been known for their consumption of yoghurt. Besides using yoghurt in cooking (one traditional favourite is a soup combining yoghurt with cucumbers), they also dilute it with water and drink it after consuming alcohol to prevent a hangover, or give it to children as a diarrhoea remedy.

### Beat Mid-day Blues

Have a yoghurt snack sometime during the day, and you'd be alert and ready to face the stresses of the day. Yoghurt contains the amino acid tyrosine, needed for the production of the neurotransmitters, dopamine and noradrenalin. Tyrosine becomes depleted when we are under stress. Thus, having some yoghurt can improve your memory and keep you alert.

### Easy Tips to Eat Yoghurt

Add cocoa powder and some sugar to your plain yoghurt to make your own non-fat chocolate-flavoured yoghurt.

Liven up the flavour of plain yoghurt by adding vanilla, almond or lemon extract, or spice it up with cinnamon, cardamom or ginger.

If you prefer savoury, add chilli, curry leaves, herbs of your choice, mustard, salsa and/or grated vegetables to the yoghurt to make a dip, or to eat as is.

Follwing are more recipes:

Fresh fruit yoghurt: Chop several types of fresh fruits (apples, grapes, mango), blend at low speed till partly liquefied and then add the yoghurt with a dash of brown sugar. Refrigerate and eat when cool.

Yoghurt banana split: Cut a banana in half lengthwise and place in a long, shallow dish. Dice three different kinds of fruit separately and pile them in three separate mounds between the banana slices. Pour yoghurt on top of the fruits and cover with more fruits or honey/maple syrup. Finish by sprinkling some nuts and wheatgerm.

Frozen yoghurt: Mix yoghurt with fruit or any flavouring and freeze it for a few hours. Thaw it slightly, and stir it up before eating it. You could also sprinkle sunflower seeds, chopped nuts or wheatgerm over flavoured yoghurt for a pleasant crunch.

Top low-fat granola cereal with yoghurt instead of milk for a delicious breakfast or afternoon snack.

Also, low-fat shakes are easy to make by blending yoghurt with fresh or frozen fruit.

## Also Try These Winning Combinations

### Yoghurt + Flaxseed

Our gut houses four hundred kinds of bacteria. Some are friendly, while others bad for us. When the bad bugs become more than the good ones, digestion becomes slow and the bowels get sluggish. Yoghurt can help get things moving again by delivering probiotics, the good-for-us bacteria. But these probiotics need to feed on another kind of probiotics—specialized fibres found in foods like flaxseed—to survive and thrive. When you eat them together, you restore and then maintain the healthy balance in the belly. It doesn't get any easier than this: Sprinkle a tablespoon of ground flaxseed over your probiotic yoghurt, season with black pepper and salt and dig in. Like it a little sweet? Dress it up a bit, and make a fruit and yoghurt parfait with flaxseed granola to add some crunch. You can get the probiotics via onions too: onion-tomato raita, anyone?

### Yoghurt + Banana

Bananas contain inulin, which fuels the growth of yoghurt's healthy bacteria. Also, this combination is cooling, so it is a boon for the summer months too. In fact, a chilled banana-yoghurt smoothie is a perfect mid-evening snack.

### Roti + Raita

Are you planning to eat wholegrain rotis tonight? By dunking it into a yoghurt-based curry or a raita, you'll ensure that the zinc is absorbed better from the grains. Eating Continental or Mediterranean? Get some wholewheat bread and tzatziki (a Greek yoghurt dip) on the side. Or simply opt for rye bread this time round, and pair it with a yoghurt smoothie.

### Yoghurt + Almonds

Your body needs the difficult-to-find vitamin D to absorb bone-building calcium better, and almond is one of the rare food sources of vitamin D, so it helps put the calcium in yoghurt to good use. Also, the fat present in yoghurt returns the favour by improving the absorption of fat-soluble vitamin D.

## At a Glance

The benefits of eating yoghurt include,

- Generating good bacteria in the gut
- Strengthening the bones
- Scoring high-quality protein
- Slowing down ageing
- Getting heart-healthy potassium

### Fun Fact
The name yoghurt was derived from the Turkish term 'yogurur', which means long life.

Mini Chapter X

## STAY COOL

**Fixit Tip 95:** To keep the body in tune with nature, always begin the day with a cooling breakfast during summers. Ragi, sattu, bajra, most lentils (especially, green moong), yoghurt, fruits and vegetables are cooling foods.

**Fixit Tip 96:** Include cooling foods like fresh ginger, marjoram, cilantro, lemon balm, peppermint and white peppercorn, and avoid cinnamon and dry ginger as they are warming.

**Fixit Tip 97:** Mint is a great appetizer; it promotes digestion, soothes summer cramps, and prevents acidity and inflammation in the stomach, all of which are common problems during summers.

**Fixit Tip 98:** During summer, have roasted barley water or buttermilk along with your meals to prevent sunstroke; they are inherently cooling.

**Fixit Tip 99:** Cucumber is the most cooling food and should be eaten more during the hot months. They are amazingly alkaline, are hydrating due to the high water content and have lignin, which helps boost our immunity as well as heart health.

**Fixit Tip 100:** Lychees are delicious, no doubt! And this sweetest of all fruits delivers vitamin C too, besides multiple hard-to-find electrolytes. So, it is a perfect fruit for beating summer blues.

# PART 2

## 10 TOOLS: FOODS TO HELP YOU BECOME HEALTHIER

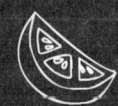

# 10 PEELS THAT YOU MUST EAT

## 1. Apple

Apple peel is loaded with a compound called quercetin, which improves lung function. It also has ursolic acid, which helps build muscle.

Eating Cue: Throw away the peeler, just scrub the fruit well and consume *with* the peel.

## 2. Orange

Orange peel is especially loaded with antioxidant hesperidin, which helps lower blood pressure and tame LDL cholesterol. Also, the compounds called polymethoxylated flavones found in these peels have the potential to lower cholesterol very effectively.

Eating Cue: Don't just throw away the peel; add the zest to your smoothies, salads, soups and stir-fries. Or brew a tea with it. You can aslo add some zest to the juice too.

## 3. Lemon

Lemon peel is loaded with dietary fibres like hemi-cellulose and pectin, which are known to stabilize blood sugar and are natural appetite suppressants. Also, the monoterpenes in citrus fruit (the oils that give oranges and lemons their special scent) help prevent skin, liver, lung and stomach cancers—and these are found mostly in the peel.

Eating Cue: Grate some lemon peel and add it to warm water; drink this for more effective weight control. Also, dry and powder the peels and add wherever possible (cakes, cookies, etc.), or just chew on them bit by bit—the taste will grow on you.

## 4. Cucumber

The peel on the cucumber is loaded with vitamin K, which helps with bone-building and maintenance. It is a good source of beta-carotene, a type of vitamin A too, which is essential for eye health.

Eating Cue: Cut it for salads with the peel.

## 5. Pear

Pear peels boost the fibre content without too much of an increase in the calories, which helps gain satiety. That's because the skin of the pear is equal to half of the pear's total dietary fibre. Pear skin has a lot of vitamin K too.

Eating Cue: Bite in without peeling it.

## 6. Potato

Potato skin is loaded with vitamin C and B6, potassium, manganese and copper.

Eating Cue: So next time you make mashed potatoes, just scrub the potatoes really well and leave the peels on.

## 7. Brinjal

Brinjal skin is loaded with anthocyanin pigments, which work overtime against cancer, ageing and inflammation. It is loaded with nasunin, an anthocyanin that boosts the brain, protects it from free radical damage and improves memory.

Eating Cue: Cook brinjal with the skin on, to improve your memory, and learn to celebrate its purple colour.

## 8. Radish

Avoid peeling the radish as the potent disease-saving antioxidant allyl isothiocyanates, which gives a peppery pungent flavour to this root vegetable, are thickly concentrated in the peel.

Eating Cue: Next time you make mooli parantha, wash the mooli properly and then grate along with the peel.

## 9. Banana

The peel of a banana is loaded with serotonin, a hormone that helps beat depression, and keeps us in a happy mood. It also delivers lutein, an antioxidant that helps the retina cells to renew.

Eating Cue: Cut the peel into small pieces and boil in water for some time. Then strain and drink the water.

## 10. Mango

Mango skin contains properties similar to resveratrol (the pigment that made wine famous), which helps burn fat and prevent insulin resistance. It also contains more carotenoids, polyphenols, Omega-3, Omega-6 and polyunsaturated fatty acids than its flesh.

Eating Cue: Chew some of the peel too when digging into a mango. Or have mango the original way (by eating the flesh off the peel, rather than chopping into cubes and eating with a fork). This way, a bit of the tangy flavour from the peels flows into the flesh too. Also, scraping the flesh from the peel gets you more of the disease-busting antioxidants that are near the peel—anthocyanins and resveratrol.

### Note:
If you are worried about pesticides and other contaminants, wash the fruits and vegetables thoroughly and then to be doubly sure, wash them with 1 part vinegar mixed with 4 parts water, wash again with cold water and then gently pat dry using a soft cloth.

II

# 5 ANCIENT GRAINS TO GET BACK ON OUR PLATE ASAP

It's time to make what's old, new again! Consciously start eating all sorts of grains with ancient pedigrees, which we have all but discarded these days. To begin with, let's aim for half our grains to be whole (and different) every day. It's not that difficult.

My list of grains to begin plating ASAP is as follows:

## 1. Amaranth

### Complete Protein

The benefits of eating amaranth (rajgira) include its delicious peppery taste and the fact that it is a brilliant source of complete protein. It contains all the essential amino acids including lysine and methionine, which are usually lacking in vegetarian protein sources.

### Low Glycemic Index

Its low glycemic index makes it great for diabetics and also for people looking to lose weight. Plus, it is gluten-free and has some peptides (the same ones that are found in soybeans), which have anti-carcinogenic and anti-inflammatory properties.

*Nutrients Load*

It is the richest source of iron and vitamin E among the grains. It is also high in calcium and a rare grain that has some vitamin C too.

Eating Cue: I love the fact that it doesn't lose its crunchiness even after being cooked, and makes for a great breakfast porridge. I often use it in place of breadcrumbs in recipes, and amaranth pops make a delicious snack.

## 2. Barley

*The Resistant Starch Advantage*

The oldest-known grain, barley (jau) is a brilliant source of resistant starch, a kind of fibre that helps lower cholesterol (yes, even more than oat fibre) and can help control blood sugar too. Resistant starch, which functions like soluble, fermentable fibre, also boosts the good bacteria on reaching the intestines, keeping our gut health in good shape.

*Nutrients Load*

Barley delivers decent calcium, potassium and vitamins B and C. It also helps in maintaining the heart's function by helping stabilize blood pressure.

Eating Cue: Add some grains regularly in soups and salads, or cook them as a side dish. I personally love a stir-fry where I pair barley with mushrooms, lots of garlic and a sauce of choice.

## 3. Buckwheat

### Protein Load

Buckwheat (kuttu) is packed with high-quality protein and offers a lot of the amino acid lysine, which is missing from most of our regular/preferred staples—wheat and rice. That's great news for vegetarians who are always struggling for good quality protein.

### Cholesterol Cutter

This is the only grain known to have a high level of an antioxidant called rutin, which improves circulation and prevents LDL cholesterol from blocking blood vessels. It is also the richest source of a unique carbohydrate, called D-chiro-inositol, which helps reduce blood sugar and prevent diabetes, and is safe for diabetics to eat too.

### Gut Helper

It contains a lot of soluble and insoluble fibre that keeps us full for long, and helps in detoxifying the body by binding to toxins and throwing them out.

### Gluten-free

It is gluten-free and so is good for people suffering from coeliac disease and also for those who voluntarily want to go on grain- and gluten-free diets.

Eating Cue: Besides kuttu roti, you can add buckwheat grains to soups and salads to score health with a dash of crunchiness.

## 4. Finger Millet

### Digestion Helper

This underrated gluten-free grain, also known as ragi, has a lot going for it. It is packed with cellulose, a type of dietary fibre that helps keep our digestion humming along, constipation away and cholesterol levels in check.

### Nutrient Load

It is a rich source of calcium and iron, and its main protein fraction, eleusinin, has a high biological value (meaning it is easily absorbed and used in the body).

### Great for Diabetics

Like barley, ragi too is an ideal food for diabetics, and overweight people because its digestion is slow and glucose is released from the intestines gradually into the blood.

Eating Cue: Add ragi idli, dosa, crêpes and ladoos to your menu and bring some life and health to it.

## 5. Pearl Millet

### Great for Monsoons

Digestion gets a little sluggish during the rainy reason, so it helps to stick to high-fibre and gluten-free foods like pearl millets (bajra). In fact, it delivers a lot of insoluble fibre that provides bulk to the stool and keeps constipation, a common problem during rains, at bay.

## Your Heart's Friend

Bajra attacks from three fronts: Its magnesium helps keep the heart healthy, potassium helps reduce the overall blood pressure, and fibre helps reduce the LDL (bad) cholesterol. Magnesium also helps control the glucose receptors in the body and keep diabetes at bay.

## A Brilliant Detoxifying Agent

Millet contains catechins like quercetin, which help keep the kidney and liver functioning properly by eliminating the toxins from the body.

Eating Cue: Smear a hot bajra roti with ghee and eat it with a little jaggery, or make bajra khichri. It is delicious!

III

# 5 SUMMER COOLERS

### 1. Green Moong Sprouts

This lentil is a great cooling agent as it cools from within.

Eating Cue: Drink the water in which green moong dal has been soaked overnight. Or eat moong sprouts for breakfast.

### 2. Kokum

It is a very cooling food and is consumed extensively in Gujarat and the Konkan region.

Eating Cue: During summers, use it as a substitute for tamarind in your cooking.

### 3. Fresh Coconut Water

Fresh coconut water is loaded with essential minerals that keep the body hydrated and maintain its electrolyte balance.

Eating Cue: Drink coconut water every evening instead of your regular tea. Or make a smoothie with it for breakfast.

### 4. Bitter Gourd

Bitter gourd (karela) takes away the heat from the body, even if you indulge in heating foods occasionally.

Eating Cue: Cook karela twice a week at least.

## 5. Bottle Gourd

This gourd is mostly water (about 96 per cent), is a cooling food and delivers potassium that helps maintain electrolyte balance and prevents fatigue during summers.

Eating Cue: Make lauki juice.

IV

# 7 STAY-HAPPY FOODS

Sometimes, feeling unhappy has nothing to do with your circumstances, but everything to do with what you are (or not) plating. Yes, there are some happy nutrients and happy foods, the deficiency of which can send you down the blue lane very quickly. And eating these foods consciously can have a very positive effect on our mood.

## 1. Banana

The reason why banana ranks as a happy food is due to the great amount of tryptophan and tyrosine it contains. They're both precursors to 'happy' neurotransmitters—serotonin and dopamine! It is also rich in potassium—a vital mineral for nerve functions, and also contains natural sugars that are quickly released into the bloodstream, making one feel energetic. It has carbs of just the right kind (which releases instant energy in the body, just when you need it).

Eating Cue: Add bananas to cold cereal, make a shake with yoghurt, eat in the late afternoon, add sliced to a fruit salad, or try a peanut butter-and-banana sandwich, topped with honey.

## 2. Turmeric

Turmeric tastes bitter but is exactly what you need to stay super-healthy and depression-free. That is, thanks to the much-feted compound curcumin in it, which helps lift the level of the neuro-chemicals, norepinephrine, dopamine and serotonin, making us happier as a result. Curcumin provides a safe and effective alternative to anti-depressant medication minus its side effects. Yes, it's that effective!

Eating Cue: Use it liberally in tadkas (temperings), add to milk, or sip turmeric-infused tea.

### 3. Walnut

Walnuts deliver mood-boosting Omega-3 fatty acids, a nutrient our body needs to fight depression. They are, in fact, a vegetarian source of Omega-3. They also deliver magnesium, another happy nutrient.

Eating Cue: Just pop in a few halves regularly before bedtime as this way, it'll help you sleep better, and good sleep is a prerequisite for staying happy.

### 4. Guava

Not many people know that guavas are loaded with vitamin C–they contain four times the vitamin C in oranges! Now, besides being an effective immune booster and an anti-ageing agent for our skin and collagen, C is an effective natural anti-depressant too. In fact, people who have vitamin C deficiency often complain of unexplained moodiness and tiredness.

Eating Cue: Snack on a guava every day when in season, and with the peel on, as the peel and the flesh just underneath its thick outer rind have exceptionally higher levels of vitamin C.

### 5. Chickpea

Both kinds of chickpeas–desi (Bengal gram or kala chana) and kabuli (safed chana) are nutrition packed. They are both loaded with 'happy mood' B vitamins: B1, or thiamine, which is important for the health of the brain and nervous system; and B9 (folate) and B6 (pyridoxin), which help the body make the happy hormones, serotonin and norepinephrine.

Eating Cue: Aim for at least half a cup of cooked chickpeas (alternating between both kinds) thrice a week at least. Besides curries, you can add them to salads and soups, or just roast them (drizzle olive oil, roast at 400°F for 30-40 minutes, and add salt) and keep handy for snacking. Also eat hummus often.

## 6. Pumpkin Seeds

These crunchy green-coloured seeds with a nutty flavour deliver iron, magnesium and zinc—minerals that influence the mood. They also deliver an amino acid called tryptophan, which help keep us calm by lowering anxiety.

Eating Cue: Try eating 1 tbsp of pumpkin seeds every day. Snack on them, or sprinkle over cereals and bhelpuri. You can also add them to your smoothies, salads, soups and traditional drinks like thandai and khus.

## 7. Fig

An excellent source of potassium and fibre, figs are a good source of vitamin B6 too, which is responsible for producing mood-boosting serotonin. It also helps lower cholesterol and prevent water retention. If you are on the pill, go on a fig overdrive as the pill depletes B6 in the body and you need an extra dosage. Fresh figs are not so easily available in our country but dried figs are in abundance, so snack on these instead.

Eating Cue: Add figs to oats and porridges, muffins, cakes and salads; eat dried figs as a healthy energy snack; or stew dried figs in fruit juice. You can even spread fig butter on toast, rice cakes or crackers. To make it, boil dried figs in fruit juice until soft, then blend in a processor until smooth.

V

# 7 FOODS THAT HELP CORRECT HORMONAL IMBALANCE

The havoc that hormones can cause is huge. Patchy skin, severe acne, excess hair on the face, debilitating fatigue, fluctuating weight, an irregular menstrual cycle, dry, brittle hair, mood swings, depression, anxiety, appetite changes, low libido, poor fertility–the symptoms of hormonal imbalance in the body and their severity may vary in different people, but they are relentless and very distressing. They are today an epidemic of sorts.

However, this hormonal chaos is not a lost cause. Even though hormones sound complex (after all, there are about 200 of them working in the body), it is not that difficult to tame them as long as you gently keep resetting them. Here, the food you eat plays a major role. To keep your hormones happy, include these 7 foods in your diet on a regular basis.

## 1. Spirulina to Tackle Estrogen

Excess of estrogen can show up as abdominal obesity, bloating, cold hands and feet, hair loss, mental fogginess, hot flashes, night sweats and temperature swings. Spirulina contains the essential fatty acids that help the liver to metabolize the excess estrogen.

Eating Cue: You can have it mixed with water or just add to smoothies.

## 2. Cinnamon to Keep Insulin Stable

Insulin regulates sugar in our body. Its imbalance results in tiredness, hunger, brain fog and weight gain. Just a pinch of cinnamon is enough to keep the blood sugar stable through the day, and insulin tamed.

Eating Cue: Add a pinch of cinnamon to your morning cup of tea or coffee.

## 3. Sesame Seeds to Keep the Thyroid Healthy

Thyroid imbalance affects our metabolism and we feel cold and sluggish all the time. Sesame seeds are great for the thyroid gland as they are a good source of selenium. Thyroid has the highest selenium content of any organ, and selenium deficiency is often the reason behind thyroid disorders.

Eating Cue: Munch on them during mid-mornings.

## 4. Banana to Increase Melatonin

Sleep problems are associated with higher weight and hormonal imbalance. This results in fatigue, impaired memory and lack of concentration. Pile on vitamin B6-rich foods, particularly banana. Banana helps the body produce melatonin, the sleep hormone, which helps you sleep well and stay rested.

Eating Cue: Just peel and bite in.

## 5. Ghee to Keep Cortisol Low

When the stress hormone cortisol rises, it encourages the conversion of blood sugar into fat for long-term storage (and our weight increases). It also causes cravings, addictions, irritability, frequent headaches, anxiety and high blood pressure. Eating ghee from grass-fed cows can help keep cortisol low.

Eating Cue: Cook at least one vegetable in some ghee, or make your dal tadka with it.

### 6. Spinach to Boost Adiponectin

This fat-burning hormone works on the brain to regulate inflammation and oxidative stress, both of which contribute to weight gain. Have spinach as it has certain enzymes and antioxidants that stimulate this hormone.

Eating Cue: Eat tender spinach leaves as part of a salad, or make spinach soup.

### 7. Jamun to Strengthen the Liver

The liver cleans out toxins that we are exposed to (works as a filter) and also produces most hormones. Jamun, also known as Java Plum, can keep it healthy as it prevents fatty liver, and the resultant multiple hormonal imbalances.

Eating Cue: Make jamun chutney, jamun squash or just snack on them.

**Note:**
All our hormones are interconnected, and interact and work together synergistically—so when one gets imbalanced, it can start a negative cascading effect. So, to keep your weight and health in check, it is important to eat a hormone-stabilizing diet.

# 8 INDIAN BERRIES WE ALL MUST EAT

## 1. Cape Gooseberry

The tarty cape gooseberry (rasbhari) is one of the most potent (and delicious) forms of vitamin C that you can eat. It is packed with antioxidants and cancer-fighting phytochemicals like anthocyanins, pelargonidins, gallic acid, cyanidins, coumaric, catechins, kaempferols, ellagic acid, ferulic acid and salicylic acid. In fact, it has an oxygen radical absorbance capacity (ORAC)—which depicts the total antioxidant capacity of a food—of 4,900 units per 100 gm, which is exceptionally high.

An unsung weight-loss superfood, it helps with losing weight thanks to its high fibre content, and also a high level of manganese that boosts the basal metabolic rate (the amount of energy we burn while at rest). Also, the natural chemical responsible for rasbhari's mouthwatering aroma is similar to capsaicin (what the hot peppers are known for) and is known to fire up metabolism.

## 2. Jamun

Jamun is a proven anti-ageing food, thanks to the multiple antioxidants it delivers. The ORAC of jamun is 2,036 units. This fruit is very low on calories and is completely fat-free, making it a perfect choice for those watching their calories. Jamun is hypoglycaemic—eating it helps keep the blood sugar stable, and this makes it a popular diabetes-preventive food.

Its high iron content makes it a must-eat food for those prone to anaemia. Jamun also helps strengthen the liver, which is our body's master filter as it cleans out toxins that we are exposed to and is the powerhouse of all hormone production and metabolism. Jamun also prevents excessive lipid accumulation, which leads to fatty liver.

## 3. Phalsa

This really tiny, dark purple berry, with a beautiful balance of sweet and sour flavours, is similar to blueberries. It is extremely rich in calcium, iron, magnesium, potassium, phosphorus and vitamin C, and also contains anthocyanin flavonoids, which protect against cancer.

It is high in potassium and low in sodium, so it's a good friend of our heart. Besides this, it also purifies the blood and regulates blood pressure and cholesterol levels.

Phalsa is a cooling food that makes it perfect for summers. It helps purify the blood and helps achieve a detoxified body and glowing skin.

## 4. Rose Apple

Also called jambul and safed jamun, this fruit usually looks like a cross between a peach and an almost-yellow mangosteen, and has a very distinct rose flavour. 100 gm of this pretty-looking fruit, which ranges from white to green to yellow to red in colour, will give you only 25 calories. Yes—it is a very weight-friendly fruit!

That's only the beginning. This modest, unassuming fruit is also a powerhouse of vitamin C (37 per cent of the daily requirement), therefore it's a great immune booster and has a good amount of heart-friendly potassium (and no sodium), which is great for keeping blood pressure down.

It has a positive effect on our pancreas too (blocks the conversion of starch into sugar), so it's absolutely great for diabetics.

Jambul is a great friend of our gut: Its juice, with a little rock salt added to it, helps cure stomach disorders like indigestion and diarrhoea, and keeps constipation away. It is very popular in Odisha and West Bengal. So, bite in whenever you find them. They make a good fruit sherbet, syrup and squash too.

## 5. Dwarf Mulberry

This berry, also known as shahtoot, is a soft, really sweet fruit, which also delivers multiple antioxidants, one of which is the famous resveratrol, which is believed to prevent cancer. Shahtoot also contain alkaloids that activate macrophages, the white blood cells that stimulate the immune system and protect us from seasonal viruses.

It has a high content of vitamin A, which strengthens our eyesight and relieves eye strain. Do you spend hours staring at the computer screen? Shahtoot will be great for you!

## 6. Karonda

This tiny, pink-coloured berry, with tiny seeds at its core, is sour but tastes delicious when eaten with a sprinkling of rock salt. Eat more of these as they are a great source of natural fibre called pectin, which helps combat high cholesterol and high triglycerides, and helps prevent colon cancer and prostate cancer.

The fruit also shows anti-diabetic potential and is a blood sugar stabilizer, besides working as a guard against liver damage.

Karonda also helps prevent anaemia as it is a good source of iron.

## 7. Kokum

Kokum is great for our digestion and cools the body during summers. It contains hydroxycitric acid, which acts as an appetite suppressant.

It is loaded with magnesium, potassium and manganese, which protect against heart disease and also aid in control of blood pressure.

Garcinol, an active constituent present in kokum, is anti-carcinogenic.

## 8. Indian Jujube

This berry, also known as ber, is mostly sweet, with a hint of sourness, and a sharp crunch to it. The high amounts of vitamins C and A in it make it a great antioxidant that also helps boost the immune system.

Rich in calcium, it helps strengthen the bones, muscles and teeth.

It can also help fight Alzheimer's by reversing cell degeneration and aiding in the cognitive functioning of the brain.

VII

# 8 HEALTHY-HAIR FOODS

Incorporating the following foods in your diet will help you to naturally take good care of your scalp and hair.

## 1. Go Nuts

Brazil nuts are one of nature's best sources of selenium, an important mineral for the health of your scalp. Walnuts contain alpha-linolenic acid, an Omega-3 fatty acid that helps condition your hair. Cashews, pecans and almonds are also terrific sources of zinc. Zinc deficiency can lead to hair shedding, so make sure nuts are a regular on your healthy-hair menu.

Eating Cue: Munch on a variety of nuts every day.

## 2. Carrot

Carrots are an excellent source of vitamin A, which promotes a healthy scalp. Since a healthy scalp is essential for a shiny, well-conditioned head of hair, you'd be wise to include carrots in your diet.

Eating Cue: Eat as snacks or toppings on your salad, or make gajar ka halwa during the winters.

## 3. Sweet Potato

Our body needs vitamin A to promote the growth of the cells and tissues of the hair and scalp. Sweet potato helps to produce healthy sebum (oil) in the scalp.

Eating Cue: Make a chaat with sweet potatoes and eat in the evenings.

### 4. Beetroot

Vitamin B6 deficiency can reduce blood and oxygen supply to the hair, leading to hair loss, damaged hair and slow regrowth. Besides this, B6 also helps create melanin, the pigment that gives hair its colour. Score B6 via beetroot.

Eating Cue: Cook this humble root more—make a subzi, or add to your vegetable juices.

### 5. Garlic

Garlic helps to regulate the thyroid hormones. A thyroid disorder is the number one cause of disease-related hair loss. Garlic is a good way to reduce it.

Eating Cue: Have two cloves every morning.

### 6. Wholegrains

Focus on wholewheat bread and fortified wholegrain breakfast cereals, for a hair-healthy dose of zinc, iron and B vitamins—a boon for your hair strands.

Eating Cue: Replace refined foods with whole foods wherever possible.

### 7. Greens

Spinach and broccoli both deliver vitamins A and C, which our body needs to produce sebum, the oily substance secreted by our hair follicles, which is the body's natural hair conditioner.

Eating Cue: Cook them by rotation two to three times a week.

## 8. Low-fat Dairy Products

Skimmed milk and yoghurt are great sources of calcium, an important mineral for hair growth.

Eating Cue: Drink and eat some low-fat dairy everyday.

VIII

# 8 WOW-SKIN FOODS

The most effective answer to staying beautiful can be found in the grocery store—in fruits, vegetables and other healthy foods that are perfect to add that glow to your face; and also keep you slim and supple. Go on, add all these to your weekly diet.

## 1. Lemon

Begin your day with some lemon juice to clean out the toxins and keep the skin blemish- and acne-free. This will also give a big boost of vitamin C to make your skin baby soft. Lemons improve bowel movement too, which keeps constipation at bay, a common cause of pimples, spots and super-oily skin.

Eating Cue: Drink lemon juice with warm water and 1 tsp honey every morning.

## 2. Wheatgrass

Wheatgrass works as a fabulous tonic for your skin. It boosts the immune system and detoxifies the blood, which reflects as healthy and glowing skin.

Eating Cue: Add to your salads and drink its freshly prepared juice.

## 3. Coconut Water

Coconut water is loaded with potassium (delivers four times more than a banana), antioxidants, and cytokines, which boost circulation, help clear the pores and make the skin lustrous. No wonder in Hawaii they call it 'Noelani'—dew from the heavens.

Eating Cue: Drink coconut water every evening.

## 4. Amla

Amla helps to detoxify the liver and aid digestion. It is also a good source of vitamin C and other minerals that are good for the skin.

Eating Cue: Make amla chutney to eat with your meals.

## 5. Wheatgerm

Wheatgerm provides the B vitamin biotin. Biotin deficiency often shows up as dry and scaly skin. It also delivers zinc, which assists in the production of new cells and helps your skin glow.

Eating Cue: Sprinkle on your salads and stir-fries liberally.

## 6. Yoghurt

Yoghurt helps in the production of collagen, which reduces signs of ageing and also delivers probiotics that help prevent acne.

Eating Cue: Have a cup of yoghurt with your lunch every day. Or snack on it in the evening paired with a fruit.

## 7. Orange

If you want to keep those wrinkles away, then eat oranges. The secret lies in its high vitamin C content (one orange meets your daily requirements), which is an effective anti-ageing antioxidant.

Eating Cue: Just peel and eat.

## 8. Walnut

Snack on these! Walnuts are a delicious and crunchy way to keep your skin young, as they are packed with skin-friendly antioxidants.

Eating Cue: Add walnuts to all your cakes and make them a part of your trail mix.

# 13 EASY FOODS THAT CAN HELP SAVE YOU FROM POLLUTION

The effect of pollution on our health is well documented. It is deadly and should not be ignored. Some foods can help reduce the harm drastically.

### 1. Apple

Apples have quercetin and khellin, which boost our lung capacity and help reduce wheezing by opening up stuffed airways.

Eating Cue: Have two apples every day.

### 2. Banana

Bananas deliver potassium, low levels of which are linked to shortness of breath; and pyridoxine (vitamin B6), which helps relax lung muscles.

Eating Cue: Include bananas in your daily diet.

### 3. Carrot

The beta-carotene in carrots keeps our lungs clear of toxins.

Eating Cue: Add carrots to subzis and vegetable juices.

### 4. Clove

Cloves help to break up phlegm in the throat and esophagus, and prevent respiratory tract infections.

Eating Cue: Use more cloves in cooking. Also place a clove under your tongue and keep sucking on it slowly, whenever you step out.

## 5. Custard Apple

Custard apples works like bananas, as they are also rich in the elusive vitamin B6; and pyridoxin, which cuts inflammation caused by the toxic air we breathe.

Eating Cue: Have more of this delicious fruit, or make a dessert with it.

## 6. Flaxseed

Flaxseeds help cut the risk of allergic reactions to pollutants, thanks to the high levels of phytoestrogens and Omega-3 fatty acids.

Eating Cue: Sprinkle some on your salads and soups.

## 7. Garlic

Allicin in garlic helps the blood vessels in the lungs work well even under the onslaught of toxic pollutants.

Eating Cue: Eat two cloves of garlic every morning.

## 8. Ginger

This helps stamp air pollutants out of the air passages before they reach and irritate the lungs.

Eating Cue: Add ginger liberally to your morning and evening cup of tea.

## 9. Grapes

The resveratrol in this juicy fruit helps cut the inflammation of the cell lining of the lungs.

Eating Cue: Eat as is, or add to your salads.

## 10. Amla

Amla delivers vitamin C that stops the damage to lung tissue caused by environmental toxins.

Eating Cue: Make a chutney with it and keep handy.

## 11. Mint

The antihistamines in mint are perfect antidotes for the side effects of pollution, like nasal congestion, mucous formation and sneezing.

Eating Cue: Make a chutney with it and keep handy.

## 12. Pineapple

The enzyme bromelin in pineapples helps clean out the lungs and detoxify them naturally.

Eating Cue: Eat a couple of slices every day.

## 13. Turmeric

Turmeric works as a tonic to relieve congestion. It helps cut respiratory ailments like cough and asthma, and the curcumin in it helps reduce inflammation (caused due to pollution) in your body.

Eating Cue: Have haldi milk every night and also add to all your tadkas.

X

# 15 SUPER CONDIMENTS

## 1. Carom Seeds

High in the chemical thymol, carom seeds increase the secretion of gastric juices and help us absorb food better. They also help ease bowel movement (as a natural laxative) and prevent as well as cure constipation. To not gain excess weight or even to knock off a few pounds, it is important that our digestive system works well, and the food we eat gets digested and eliminated properly. The seeds also helps in treating a cold, clearing nasal blockage and warding off flu, besides helping deal with respiratory ailments like asthma and bronchitis and providing relief from a migraine headache.

Eating Cue: Just eat 2 gm of pan-roasted ajwain seeds every day. Or you can have ajwain tea (boil water, add black or green tea, ajwain, ginger and elaichi).

## 2. Asafoetida

Asafoetida is an age-old medicine for stomach problems including gas, bloating, irritable bowel syndrome and flatulence. It also helps in relieving chest congestion and releasing phlegm. It is a natural blood thinner and helps in lowering blood pressure. It is power-packed with coumarin, a compound that aids in improving blood flow, thereby preventing the formation of clots.

Eating Cue: Add to all your tadkas, especially the too-difficult-to-digest lentils.

## 3. Coriander Seeds

Coriander seeds help control blood sugar, cholesterol and free radical production. They help lower levels of total LDL 'bad' cholesterol, while actually increasing levels of HDL 'good' cholesterol. Coriander seeds may also be particularly useful in combating carcinogens.

Eating cue: Add to all tadkas.

## 4. Coconut Milk

Coconut milk is lactose-free and so, it is okay for those with lactose intolerance. It is a popular choice with vegans too, who usually follow dairy-free diets. It has a lot of fat (about 90 per cent) and most of it is in the form of the much-maligned saturated fatty acids, but the kind that coconut milk has—the medium-chain saturated triglyceride (MCT)—goes directly to the liver, where it is rapidly metabolized and is less likely to be stored as fat. MCTs actually help reduce appetite and decrease our calorie intake, so it could actually work as a weight-loss tool. It also helps tame blood pressure because it delivers a lot of trace minerals like manganese, copper, magnesium and phosphorous, which control blood flow and keep blood vessels flexible and free from plaque build-up. Coconut milk has lauric acid, a type of MCT that helps bring bad cholesterol down and the good one up. The selenium contained in it helps keep joint inflammation away and so it works great for those prone to arthritis.

Eating Cue: While being added to curries is how it gets to be a part of our diet, some other ways of experimenting with coconut milk are by adding a few tablespoons to our coffee, having a smoothie once in a while, or whisking it and adding it to a fruit salad (try over papaya, tastes delish!).

## 5. Cumin Seeds

Cumin seeds are a very good source of iron, a mineral that is important for energy production and metabolism, and to keep your immune system healthy. Cumin helps stimulate the secretion of pancreatic enzymes, which are necessary for proper digestion and nutrient-assimilation. They have anti-carcinogenic and anti-diabetic properties as they helps enhance the liver's detoxification enzymes and work as an effective regenerative tonic for the liver and pancreas. They also work as a sedative to relieve insomnia.

Eating Cue: Add to every tadka or have cumin water (soak 1 tbsp cumin seeds in water overnight; boil, strain, cool and sip).

## 6. Curry Leaves

These slightly alkaline leaves—they are also called 'sweet neem'—add a depth to the flavour of just about anything. They have strong anti-diabetic properties as well. Curry leaves can control blood sugar levels. They protect from heart disease—increasing the 'good' cholesterol and also help with digestion. They accelerate hair growth and prevent skin infections and are even said to be instrumental in weight loss!

Eating Cue: Add it to every tadka, whether or not the recipe demands it. Also chew a few leaves early in the morning.

## 7. Saffron

Saffron (kesar) contains a dark orange, water-soluble carotene called crocin, which helps protect against cancer and is responsible for much of saffron's golden colour. Crocin also promotes learning and memory retention and protects against Parkinson's.

Eating Cue: Add saffron to desserts, or add to boiling milk.

## 8. Fenugreek Seeds

Fenugreek seeds help balance blood sugar in diabetics, as it helps decrease the insulin response. The fibre content of fenugreek extract plays a role in its ability to moderate the metabolism of glucose in the digestive tract. They are also hypolipidemic, that is, they reduce body triglycerides and serum cholesterol. They are an expectorant, laxative and anti-inflammatory, and an effective stomach tonic that helps keep colic flatulence, dysentery and diarrhoea at bay. Fenugreek seeds also help beat water retention as they are diuretic.

Eating Cue: Add the seeds to dal tadkas. Or have methi dana water (soak 1 tbsp methi seeds in water overnight; boil, cool and sip; chew the seeds).

## 9. Garlic

Garlic has sulphide compounds that reduce cholesterol, prevent and remove clots and help clear out clogged arteries. Just 2 cloves a day work wonders.

Eating Cue: Simply pop two crushed pods every morning. Or make garlic-flavoured oil (infuse pressed garlic in olive oil) and add to all soups, curries and dips.

## 10. Ginger

Ginger boosts the immune system and keeps colds and flus away. It provides pain relief from migraine headaches by blocking prostaglandins (which stimulate muscle contractions), controlling inflammation in the blood vessels and impacting some hormones.

Eating Cue: To make ginger tea, steep one or two ½-inch slices of fresh ginger in a cup of hot water. Or you could also combine ginger, soy sauce, olive oil and garlic to make a wonderful salad dressing.

## 11. Sesame Seeds

Sesame seeds are packed with lignans, which enhance the function of liver enzymes that break down fat. Plus, the essential fatty acids and protein in them help further by increasing the metabolic rate.

Eating Cue: Add to every tadka and also sprinkle roasted seeds on salads and soups.

## 12. Fennel Seeds

Fennel seeds facilitate digestion and reduce flatulence. It is an active carminative agent and helps release gas from the intestines. These seeds work as a natural diuretic, help clear out excess uric acid in the blood stream, break down bile and also promote digestion of fats in the liver. They're loaded with minerals, many of which are trace minerals that are difficult to find: copper, potassium, phosphorus, calcium, zinc, manganese, iron, selenium and magnesium. In fact, the high concentration of iron and histamine in fennel make it a good natural remedy for anaemia, as they help increase the formation of haemoglobin in the body.

Eating Cue: I add a few seeds to my morning cup of tea; this way I do away with the need to sweeten my cuppa with sugar. Try it; you'll like the mild sweetness it adds to tea. Also add the powder to veggies liberally.

## 13. Turmeric

Turmeric could aid in fat metabolism and weight loss. 'Turmeric for being trim' sounds good! Turmeric is aromatic and a stimulant. It works as a tonic to relieve congestion. It has a soothing effect on respiratory ailments such as cough and asthma. The curcumin in turmeric also acts directly on fat cells, pancreatic cells, kidney cells and muscle cells, to reduce inflammation and prevent (in fact, even reverse) insulin resistance. Curcumin helps in detoxifying the liver as well. It also prevents alcohol and other toxins from being converted into compounds that are harmful for the liver.

Eating Cue: Solid reasons to have haldi doodh at night and add to all the tadkas.

## 14. Nigella Seeds

These seeds, also called kalonji, contain the essential ingredient, thymoquinone, which helps to fight against the inflammation that builds up within the lungs due to pollution.

Eating Cue: Sprinkle kalonji liberally on dal, vegetables and even chapatti to get the benefit

## 15. Cinnamon

Sprinkling just a pinch of cinnamon on your morning tea can keep your metabolism up and blood sugar stable through the day. This helps prevent diabetes too. It can also help combat colds, flu and digestive problems.

Cinnamon has compounds called proanthocyanidin and cinnamaldehyde, which help in processing information better, which means a sharper and more efficient brain.

Eating Cue: Make cinnamon tea—add ¼ tsp of powdered cinnamon to a cup of boiling water, and steep for 10 to 20 minutes. You can also add the powder to all your bakes.

# PART 3

# 40 DELICIOUS RECIPES

# MAGNIFICENT MAINS

## Raw Papaya Subzi

Heat 1 tsp of oil in a pan, add ½ tsp mustard seeds, 2 whole red chillies, a few curry leaves, ½ tsp turmeric and chilli powder, 400 gm grated raw papaya and salt to taste. Stir-fry and add 1 tbsp lemon juice. Garnish with some coriander leaves, 2 tbsp grated coconut and 2 tbsp roasted peanuts.

## Soya Nuggets with Spinach

Wash and chop 500 gm spinach leaves and keep aside. Heat oil in a pan, add 150 gm chopped onion, and 1 tbsp ginger paste and garlic paste. After the onion turns light brown, add 150 gm chopped tomatoes, cook well, then add 100 gm soya granules and stir well. Add the spinach leaves, ½ tsp turmeric powder, ½ tsp red chilli powder and salt to taste. Add a cup of water, mix well and cover with a lid. After the granules are cooked, add ¼ tsp garam masala and ½ tsp coriander powder, and cook till the water almost evaporates. Remove from flame and eat hot with rotis.

## Guava Curry

Heat 10 ml oil, add a pinch of mustard seeds and asafoetida. Add a mix of 10 gm coriander powder, 10 gm cumin seeds, 5 gm red chilli powder and 5 gm turmeric powder diluted with a tablespoon of water. Add 500 gm guava chopped into pieces and stir-fry for 5 minutes. Add 50 gm chopped tomato and stir-fry further for 5 minute on slow heat. Add 1 tbsp sugar, salt to taste, and 10 ml lemon juice. Take off the flame and keep it covered for 2 minutes. Garnish with a chopped green chilli and fresh coriander.

## Turnips and Potatoes au Gratin

Preheat oven to 375°F. Toss together 4 cups of sliced turnips and potatoes each, peeled and thinly sliced, 1 medium onion peeled and finely sliced with 2 tbsp melted butter, and place in a 9-inch baking dish. Cover tightly and place in a preheated oven for 30 minutes. In a small pot on top of the stove, combine ½ cup milk, ⅛ tsp grated nutmeg, ¼ tsp ground white pepper, ½ tsp salt, and bring to a boil. Immediately mix in ¼ cup grated cheese. Pour milk over the potatoes and again sprinkle ¼ cup grated cheese. Replace in oven, uncovered, for another 20 to 25 minutes. When the gratin turns golden brown, it's ready to be served.

## Red Cabbage Thoran

Heat 5 ml oil in a pan, add ½ an onion and 2 green chillies chopped, 2–3 curry leaves, a few mustard seeds, 2 whole red chillies (dried) and 200 gm chopped red cabbage. Sauté till the cabbage is soft and cooked (about 8–10 minutes). Season with ½ tsp salt, and garnish with 30 gm grated coconut.

## Herbed Lentils with Spinach and Tomatoes

Take the lentils—200 gm black masoor dal and 100 gm yellow moong dal—and soak in cold water for one hour. Chop ½ a small onion and a few coriander leaves, blanch 50 gm spinach and cut half a tomato into thin slices. Dice a quarter each of a red and yellow bell pepper. Boil the dals till the mix gets nice and soft. Drain and keep it in the refrigerator. Make a dressing with 1 tbsp lemon juice, 1 tbsp olive oil, 1 tsp mustard paste and 1 tsp sugar. Toss the lentils with the cut vegetables and add the dressing. Season and eat chilled or warm.

## BREADS AND GRAINS

### Barley Salad

Combine 1 cup barley, 1.5 cups water and a pinch of salt in a pan, bring to a boil, reduce the heat and simmer till the barley gets tender (for about 45 minutes). Drain in a colander and let it cool. Combine ½ cup cherry tomatoes, ¼ cup olives, 1 tbsp mint and ½ a sliced red bell pepper in a bowl. Add the cooled barley. Whisk together 1 tbsp red wine vinegar and 1 tbsp olive oil in a small bowl and season with salt and pepper to taste. Now dress the salad and toss.

### Bajra Pongal

Slightly dry roast 70 gm broken bajra (for about 5–7 minutes). Pressure cook 30 gm green gram dal, the roasted broken bajra (the ratio of the bajra to dal should be 70:30), and salt, with 3 cups of water, till soft. Heat 1 tbsp ghee and add a few cashews. When slightly golden brown, add ½ tsp cumin seeds, ¼ tsp pepper, a few curry leaves and ½ tsp ginger paste and add it to the pongal. Have it with chhach (buttermilk).

### Amaranth Pancake

Mix ½ cup amaranth flour, 100 ml soy milk, 2 tbsp desiccated coconut, salt, a pinch of baking powder and water (if needed) and mix well. Add 1 tbsp of honey and a bit of cinnamon powder. Now heat a nonstick frying pan, add ½ a tsp of olive oil and add a dollop of the pancake mix. Spread evenly to give a round shape. Cook both sides on slow heat. Drizzle some honey on top and enjoy.

## Mixed Veg Pulao (with Brown Rice; Oil-free)

Dry roast ½ tsp jeera, add 50 gm each of chopped mushrooms and bell peppers and stir-fry dry; wait till they are a little soft. Put in 50 gm steamed broccoli, stir-fry dry till the jeera coats the veggies. Add 1 cup boiled brown rice, stir in salt to taste, and add some sliced green chillies. Remove from the flame, and add some roasted peanuts and sesame seeds.

## Sattu Parantha (Makuni Roti)

Take sattu flour. In some mustard oil, add 1 grated onion and ginger, and some amchoor, salt and chilly powder. Mix well and shape into lemon-sized balls. Flatten a tomato-sized ball of wholewheat dough into a thin disc. Place the sattu ball in the centre, gather the edges of the dough and pinch together, sealing in the sattu ball. Press gently into a thick disc and flatten into a thin sheet. Cook both sides on a hot skillet. Have it with curd.

## Masala Dosa (Made with Brown Rice)

To make the dosa, soak brown rice and washed urad dal in a 3:1 proportion, along with 1 tsp methi seeds, in a small bowl. Keep for 6 hours, and then drain the water. Grind this mixture, adding enough water to make a batter with thick consistency. Leave to ferment overnight or 6-8 hours. In a tawa, add a little oil. Put one small cup/ladle full of batter on the heated tawa and spread it into a circular shape. After this, reduce to medium heat and cover with a lid to steam for 2-3 minutes or till the underside of the dosa is brown and leaves the tawa easily.

## For the Filling

Steam 2 potatoes, chop and keep aside. Roast 1 tsp mustard seeds till they begin to pop and add 3 tbsp of water. Sauté 1 sliced onion and 2 pods of garlic in the water. When done, add 1 chopped tomato and cook till it has a thick consistency. Add salt to taste and the potatoes. Mix thoroughly and use as filling for the dosa.

### Ragi Idli

Wash and soak ½ cup urad dal and 1 cup rice separately overnight. Next day, grind both of them separately. Mix the ground rice and dal. Add ½ cup ragi flour to the mixture. Add salt to taste. Set aside for 5-6 hours for fermentation.

Steam small portions of the mixture in an idli steamer garnished with chopped vegetables. The leftover batter can go in the fridge and be used later. Eat with tomato chutney.

### Ragi Crêpe

Combine 100 gm bell peppers diced finely, 100 gm grated carrot, 100 gm chopped tomato, 100 gm chopped onion, and 2 tbsp coriander chopped finely in a bowl. Mix 1 cup ragi flour with water and make a batter, add salt, 1 tsp ginger-garlic paste, 2 chopped green chillies and mix well. Heat a griddle or nonstick pan, and brush lightly with oil. Holding the pan in one hand, pour ¼ cup batter onto the pan while rotating it so that a thin layer of batter covers the surface. Return the pan to heat and allow the crêpe to cook for 2-3 minutes or until the upper surface has dried up and the bottom is lightly browned. Place 1 tbsp chopped vegetables on the crêpe, gently spread it and cover the pan with a lid to enable the vegetables to cook well in the steam. Repeat until all the batter is used, keeping the cooked crêpes warm. Eat warm.

### Phal-ahaar

Wash about 50 gm flattened rice (½ cup chivda), drain and set aside while you peel and chop a fruit or two and gather up some nuts. Then mix it all up with 1 cup yoghurt (about 200 gm). You can also add jaggery for flavour.

### Shewaya Upma

Heat 1 tsp oil and add 1 tsp each of chana dal, urad dal, mustard seeds and a few curry leaves. As they crackle, add 2 tsp of peanuts and cashew nuts and fry a bit. Now add ½ diced potato and carrot, and after frying for 4-5 minutes, add 1 chopped chilli, grated ginger, ½ onion, some peas and ½ diced tomato, and cook till done. Now add salt and 1 cup of water, and cover with a lid. When the water comes to a boil, add ½ cup of vermicelli and stir. Cover with a lid for 5-6 minutes and the upma's done!

### Ragi Porridge

Take about 2 litres of water and boil. Slowly add 100 gm ragi powder to the boiling water, stirring constantly with a big spoon. Keep boiling until it forms a medium-thick consistency. Add salt, stir and turn off the flame. Add a bit of lemon juice and salt to 200 ml buttermilk. Now add this buttermilk to the thick ragi mix, and enjoy. You can also add a lime pickle on the side.

### Keera Puttu

Mix a small bowl of red ragi flour, 100 gm spinach and water together, and make small balls of this mixture. Add

2 chopped green chillies, ½ a cut onion, salt to taste and 2 tbsp grated coconut. Steam in either a puttu steamer or a pressure cooker without weight.

### Poitabhat

Add water to 1 cup cooked rice, cover it and leave it to ferment overnight (keep the dish covered to avoid contamination). Next morning for breakfast, add ½ an onion chopped, 2 chopped green chillies and salt to taste. Squeeze in some lemon juice. You can have this dish with a little roasted brinjal or mashed potato (other options can be achaar, various boiled veggies, dal or curries that may be leftover from the previous night). You can even have a little sour curd on the side.

### Chilled Red Rice with a Tadka

Heat 2 tbsp oil in a pan, add 1 tsp mustard seeds and 1 tsp urad dal and sauté them. Add a few curry leaves. Remove this tadka from the pan and keep aside. Take a mixing bowl and mix 250 gm yoghurt along with salt and cumin, and mix thoroughly. Add in boiled red rice and ½ a diced cucumber, and add in the prepared tadka. Refrigerate and serve cold, garnished with fried curry leaves.

## SNACK ATTACK

### Beans-and-Veggies Spread

Mash 1 small bowl of boiled rajma or lobia and mix with 1 small bowl of low-fat plain yoghurt. Add condiments as desired (mustard, dill, parsley, garlic, onion or pepper). Chill and spread it on multigrain bread and top with lettuce, sliced cucumber and tomato.

## Seasoned Sprouts

Heat 1 tbsp mustard oil. Drop ¼ tsp mustard seeds, ¼ tsp cumin, 2 chillies slit, and a pinch of asafoetida (in that order). Immediately add the sprouts and stir-fry for about 2 minutes. Add ¼ tsp sugar and stir for a minute. Turn off the heat. Add lime juice and salt to taste. Season with chopped coriander when still hot.

## Dal Patty

Grind 1 small bowl of soaked chana dal. To this, add ½ a finely chopped onion, spices (red chilli powder, coated cumin) salt, and a binder like ½ a boiled potato or some steamed cauliflower. Shape this mixture into a patty and air fry.

# HEALTHY DESSERTS

## Apple Crunch

Peel and grate 2 apples. Spread them in a baking dish. Sprinkle 2 tsp sugar, 2 tsp roasted amaranth, and a pinch of cinnamon powder over it. Bake in a medium oven for 5-6 minutes or till the apples are done.

## Parippu Payasam

Roast 100 gm parippu (yellow moong dal) without oil for 5-6 minutes. Then cook with boiled water. Melt 150 gm jaggery by adding ½ cup of water. Now add the melted jaggery to the well-cooked parippu and stir well. Add 1 tbsp ghee and mix well. Add 125 ml coconut milk and boil it. When the mix evaporates and reduces to half, remove from the stove. For the garnish, fry a few cashew nuts and coconut pieces in 1 tsp ghee and add to the payasam. Serve hot.

### Grapes Parfait

Place a few grapes at the bottom of tall, stemmed glasses. Top with 2 tbsp of sour cream, then ½ tsp of brown sugar. Repeat until the glass is filled to the desired level. Garnish with a single grape on top.

### Orange Peel Candy

Make a syrup with 2 cups water and ½ cup sugar. Bring to a boil, add the rinds of 5 oranges, and let them cook for 30 minutes on a low flame. Remove from heat, let them cool, place on wax paper and let them dry.

## SPECTACULAR SIDES

### Green Heaven

Boil spinach and chop it finely with a pair of kitchen scissors. Mix into a bowl of thick yoghurt. Temper with ½ tsp of mustard seeds and 2 green chillies in a spoon of oil. The taste is divine.

### Cucumber Raita

Mix grated cucumber with curd, fresh mint leaves, turmeric powder, roasted jeera powder and 1 tsp mashed mustard seeds.

### Curry Leaves Chutney

Take 1 tsp mustard seeds, 2 tsp curry leaves, ¼ cup chopped onions, 2 tsp crushed garlic, 1 tsp chopped green chillies, 2 tsp tamarind pulp, 1 tsp powdered sugar, salt to taste and grind them to a fine paste.

## Spicy Watermelon Salsa

In a serving bowl, mix together ½ a large watermelon (seeds removed and coarsely chopped), ½ chopped red onion, 1 red chilli (seeds removed and chopped), a handful of chopped coriander leaves, 2 tbsp balsamic vinegar and ¼ tsp salt. Cover and refrigerate for at least 1 hour.

## Cinnamon-flavoured Apple Butter

Wash 2 apples, but do not peel. Cut into small chunks and simmer in 1 cup of water until soft. Then press them through a sieve. Now heat the apple pulp in a large pan, adding ¼ cup sugar, ¼ tsp cinnamon and a pinch of clove powder. Cook slowly, stirring, until you have a thick puree that sticks to a wooden spoon without dripping. Seal in a sterilized jar. Eat with crackers or wholewheat bread.

## Sesame Salt

Mix 5 parts roasted and powdered sesame seeds with 1 part salt, and use as a flavouring. It adds an interesting flavour to food.

## Lentil Hummus

Just mix up ½ a small bowl of boiled, mashed dal (any), 1 tbsp tahini (a paste made from ground, toasted sesame seeds), garlic, a pinch of red pepper flakes, a pinch of salt and 1 tsp olive oil. Perfect on a toast!

## Peanut Butter

Grind ½ cup roasted peanuts. Add 1.5 tbsp peanut oil gradually to give it a smooth texture and grind again. Add a pinch of salt and sugar to give it a sweet-salty taste.

Put this mixture in a sealed container and refrigerate. It'll easily last for two weeks, and that too minus any unhealthy preservatives.

### Chickpea Hummus

Soak 1.5 cups of chickpeas for 4-5 hours and then pressure cook for 2-3 whistles (till they become soft enough to grind in a mixer/grinder). Cool and grind them with 3 garlic cloves, 1 tsp cumin powder, ½ tsp red chilli powder, ¼ cup sesame seeds and salt to taste. Add 1 tbsp lemon juice and 1 tbsp olive oil. Mix and set aside.

### Walnut and Herb Dip

Take ½ cup walnuts, 1 cup hung curd, a few sprigs of mint, a few sprigs of coriander, a couple of garlic flakes , and salt and pepper to taste. Blend all the ingredients into a paste. It's perfect with veggie sticks as well as crackers.

### Flaxseed Chutney

Grind together 250 gm roasted flaxseeds, a palmful of dried red chillies, and 1-2 whole garlics (the whole thing). Add salt to taste.

### Ash Gourd Chutney

Peel 250 gm ash gourd (petha) and chop the peels finely. Boil in 200 ml water till soft and then grind with 2 tbsp grated coconut, 2 fried green chillies, 1 tbsp lemon juice and 10 gm ginger.

# ACKNOWLEDGEMENTS

I want to thank a lot of people, but I will begin by thanking all the editors I have worked with across different media houses over the years. The list is really long and I am indebted to each one of them for everything they have taught me over the years. I was so raw when I began and they shaped my writing, and helped me get better with each successive stint. Some of them are dear, dear friends today, and I love them all.

To the entire team of Rupa for their support and advice, for editing the book so well, and of course, continuing to have faith in my ideas.

To my agent Anuj Bahri of Redink, for relentlessly championing my writing and showcasing my books so brilliantly.

To all my friends who love me and encourage me selflessly. I love you back. And more.

To my husband Bhanu and my son Vimanyu, who are my world.

To my sister Punita and her family for just being there for me all the time.

To all my adorable nephews and nieces—love you all!

And of course, as always to my parents, whom I love and respect immensely.